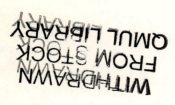

ATLAS OF
ENDOCRINE IMAGING

The picture used on the front cover is of a sellar/suprasellar macroadenoma of the pituitary, visualised by sagittal T1–weighted MR imaging.

ATLAS OF
ENDOCRINE IMAGING

EDITED BY

G Michael Besser MD DSc FRCP
Professor of Endocrinology
Physician in Charge
Department of Endocrinology
St Bartholomew's Hospital
London, UK

Michael O Thorner MB BS DSc FRCP
Kenneth R Crispell Professor of Medicine
Chief, Division of Endocrinology and Metabolism
Director, General Clinical Research Center
Department of Medicine
Health Sciences Center
University of Virginia
Charlottesville
Virginia, USA

FOREWORD BY

Professor Peter Armstrong MB BS FRCR
Head of Department of Radiology
St Bartholomew's Hospital
London, UK

ᴎ WOLFE

London St. Louis Baltimore Boston Chicago Philadelphia Sydney Toronto

For full details of all Mosby Europe Limited titles please write to: Mosby Europe Limited, Brook House, 2–16 Torrington Place, London WC1E 7LT, UK

Publisher: Fiona Foley

Project Manager: Richard French

Design: Louise Bond

Illustration: Lee Smith

Index: Nina Boyd

Production: Susan Bishop

British Library Cataloguing in Publication Data:
Library of Congress Cataloging in Publication Data:
Catalogue records for this title are available

ISBN: 1-56375-583-1

Originated in Hong Kong by Mandarin Offset (H.K.) Ltd.

Produced by Imago Productions

Printed and bound in Singapore

Text set in Garamond; figures and legends set in Futura by Colour Bytes, London

CONTRIBUTORS

Jamshed B Bomanji MD MSc PhD
Consultant Physician
Department of Nuclear Medicine

Keith E Britton MD MSc FRCP
Consultant in Charge
Department of Nuclear Medicine

Janet E Dacie FRCP DMRD FRCR
Consultant Radiologist

St Bartholomew's Hospital
London, UK

Victor M Haughton MD
Professor of Radiology
Director of Neuroradiology Research

Leighton P Mark MD
Consultant Radiologist

Robert J Witte MD
Consultant Radiologist

Medical College of Wisconsin
Froedtert Memorial Lutheran Hospital
Milwaukee
Wisconsin, USA

F Elizabeth White MRCP DMRD FRCR
Consultant Radiologist
Royal Liverpool University Hospital
Liverpool, UK

CONTENTS

FOREWORD

It is often said that a picture is worth a thousand words, and this remark is particularly true of diagnostic imaging. This atlas, which brings together a unique collection of X-rays, angiograms, CT and MRI scans, ultrasound and nuclear medicine images will, I am sure, be of enormous value to all those who see patients with endocrine disease.

The imaging of endocrine disorders crosses the dividing lines between conventional specialist divisions. Not only does it require the expert knowledge normally associated with subjects such as neuroradiology and skeletal radiology, but it also involves many different imaging modalities, often in the same patient. Nuclear medicine imaging may be used to define the sites of one or more endocrine tumours, prior to detailed anatomical imaging with ultrasound, computed tomography or MRI. Specialist angiographic techniques may also be needed, particularly for selective venous sampling. This book will, therefore, be welcomed by a wide variety of radiologists, many of whom may be called upon to investigate a patient with an endocrine disorder.

I was particularly pleased to be asked to write this foreword because I have had the rare opportunity of working with both of the editors of the companion volume, *Clinical Endocrinology*. I worked closely with Michael Thorner during my many years at the University of Virginia, and more recently have been able to observe the outstanding clinical service provided by Michael Besser.

Professor Peter Armstrong
London, England

PREFACE

The immensely dramatic advances in the understanding of human endocrine physiology over the last two decades has led to equally spectacular improvements in clinical endocrine practice. It is usual to associate these developments principally with the introduction of new methods for the simple, precise and sensitive assay of an increasing number of hormones in body fluids, under basal and dynamic conditions. While, undoubtedly, these technical advances have played a key role in allowing a sophisticated assessment of the endocrine milieu in health and disease, other changes have contributed an equal, if less heralded, part; particularly so for advances in imaging in endocrine diseases. Thus, endocrine radiological developments have been extraordinary. We can now, with combinations of magnetic resonance and computerised tomographic imaging, often with angiography, venous sampling and even still conventional radiology, visualise and confirm the functional aberrations of a large variety of disordered endocrine glands. The related nuclear imaging provides the specific and sensitive association of anatomical location and functional disturbance. We have, therefore, assembled this short book to bring together the latest information on general endocrine radiology, neuroradiology and nuclear medicine endocrine imaging, from authors widely acknowledged in their fields. We hope that it will help the interacting roles of radiologists, nuclear medicine physicians and clinical endocrinologists in reaching a conclusion in any functional disturbance in patients suspected of endocrine disease, whether rare or common. We believe that others will benefit by bringing together the commonality of these authors' wide experience.

We wish also to acknowledge the enormous help and contribution made by our colleagues Patrick Purcell, of the Department of Endocrinology at Saint Bartholomew's Hospital, and Richard French at Gower Medical Publishing, in the development of this project.

Michael Besser   Michael O Thorner
London, England   Charlottesville, USA

ACKNOWLEDGEMENTS

For the kind provision of some of the ultrasound and CT images we would like to thank Drs AT Carty, HML Carty and CJ Garvey, and for kind provision of Figure 1.23, Professor P Armstrong. Figure 1.20 was reproduced from White FE, White MC, Drury PL, Kelsey Fry I, Besser GM, *Value of computed tomography of the abdomen and chest in the investigation of Cushing's syndrome.* British Medical Journal 1982; 284: 771–4. Courtesy of the British Medical Journal, London.

1

Radiology of Endocrine Disease

Janet E Dacie, FRCP, DMRD, FRCR • F Elizabeth White, MRCP, DMRD, FRCR

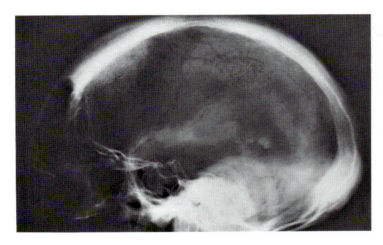

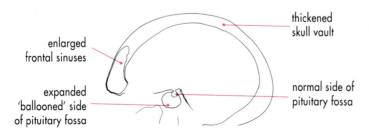

enlarged
frontal sinuses

expanded
'ballooned' side
of pituitary fossa

thickened
skull vault

normal side of
pituitary fossa

Fig.1.1 Acromegaly: lateral skull film showing vault changes and a 'ballooned' pituitary fossa. The main role of radiology in the assessment of acromegaly is to confirm the presence of a pituitary tumour and to provide information necessary for treatment and follow-up. (See Chapter 2 for a discussion of pituitary tumours.) Certain characteristic systemic changes do,however, occur in acromegaly and this lateral skull film demonstrates typical diffuse hyperostosis of the calvarium and abnormally large frontal sinuses. A double floor to the pituitary fossa can be seen. One side is of normal calibre and the other is grossly expanded i.e. 'ballooned'. (See Fig. 1.3 for details.)

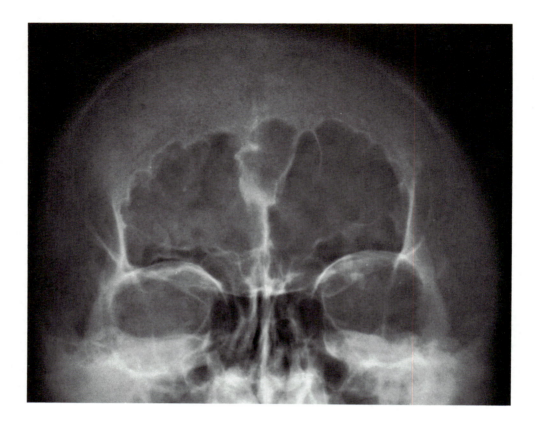

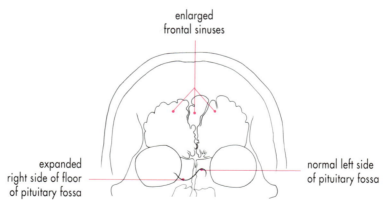

enlarged
frontal sinuses

expanded
right side of floor
of pituitary fossa

normal left side
of pituitary fossa

Fig. 1.2 Acromegaly: postero-anterior (PA) skull film showing enlarged frontal sinuses. This PA skull film of the same patient as in Fig. 1.1 demonstrates the marked enlargement of the frontal sinuses. The floor of the pituitary fossa is seen to be grossly enlarged on the right side by a large but asymmetric pituitary tumour.

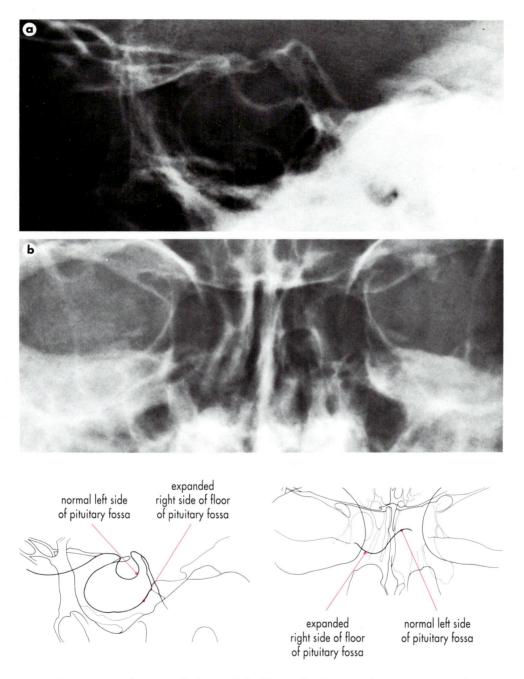

Fig. 1.3 Acromegaly: coned views of 'ballooned' pituitary fossa. These coned lateral (a) and PA (b) views of the pituitary fossa are of the same patient as in Figs. 1.1 and 1.2. They demonstrate more clearly the gross asymmetric expansion of the right side of the floor of the pituitary fossa.

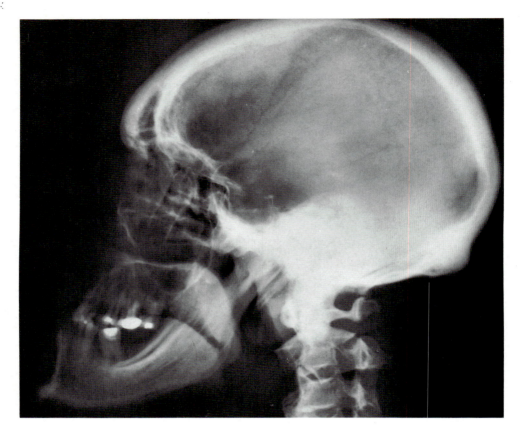

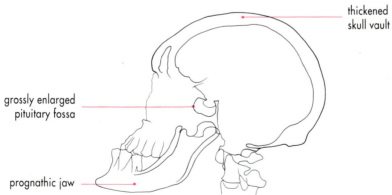

thickened
skull vault

grossly enlarged
pituitary fossa

prognathic jaw

Fig. 1.4 Acromegaly: prognathic jaw. The lateral skull film of another patient shows characteristic prognathism with increase in the normal angle of the mandible. The pituitary fossa is grossly enlarged and the skull vault is markedly thickened, particularly anteriorly, although in this patient the frontal sinuses are not enlarged.

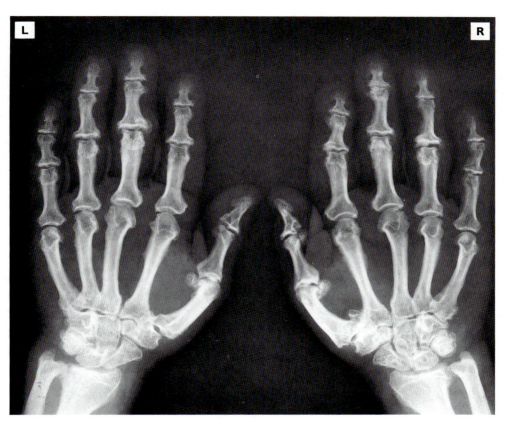

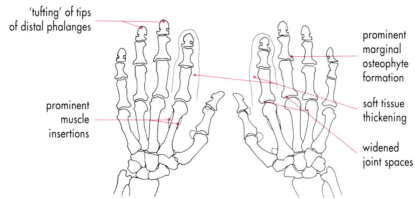

'tufting' of tips of distal phalanges

prominent marginal osteophyte formation

prominent muscle insertions

soft tissue thickening

widened joint spaces

Fig. 1.5 Acromegaly: hands. In acromegaly the hands are large and the classical radiological features include generalised soft tissue thickening, widening of the joint spaces due to hypertrophy of the articular cartilages, prominent muscle insertions particularly along the metacarpal shafts, tufting of the tips of the terminal phalanges and prominent osteophyte formation. In addition, in this patient, degenerative cysts are present in some of the carpal bones, particularly in the right carpus.

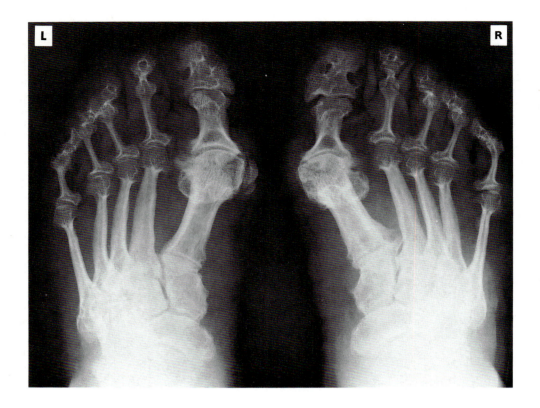

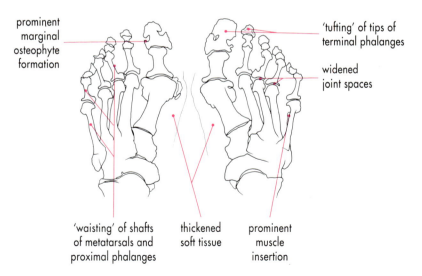

prominent
marginal
osteophyte
formation

'tufting' of tips of
terminal phalanges

widened
joint spaces

'waisting' of shafts
of metatarsals and
proximal phalanges

thickened
soft tissue

prominent
muscle
insertion

Fig. 1.6 Acromegaly: feet. The radiological changes in the hands in acromegaly are also seen in the feet but, in addition to new bone formation, bone resorption occurs giving rise to typically thinned metatarsals. Thinning of the shafts of the phalanges may also occur, as in this patient.

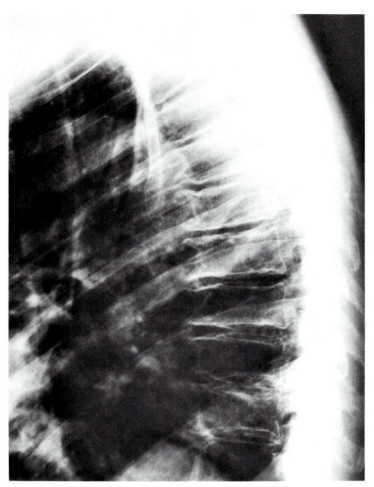

Fig. 1.7
Acromegaly:
lateral dorsal spine.

In acromegaly new bone formation may occur around the vertebral bodies. This lateral view of the dorsal spine shows such changes at the anterior margins of the vertebrae. The anterior edge of the intervertebral discs can be clearly identified and the vertebral bodies are increased in their anteroposterior diameter. The new bone formation is usually more marked in the dorsal than in the lumbar spine.

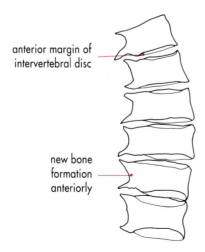

anterior margin of
intervertebral disc

new bone
formation
anteriorly

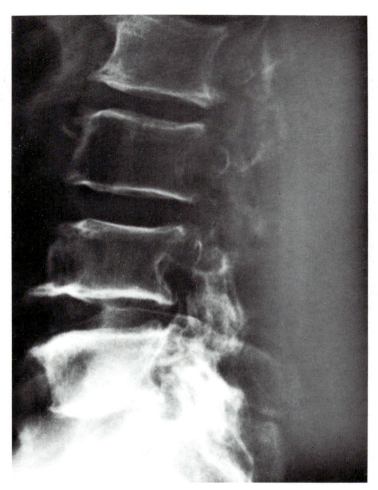

Fig. 1.8
Acromegaly:
lateral lumbar
spine. In addition to
new bone formation
anteriorly this lateral
view of the lumbar spine
shows prominent
marginal osteophyte
formation and
characteristic scalloping
of the posterior margins
of the vertebral bodies.
Although such
scalloping may be seen
in the dorsal spine, the
lumbar spine is most
commonly affected.

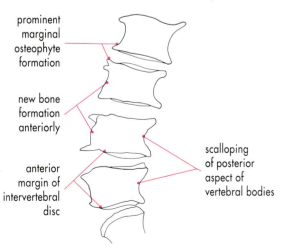

prominent
marginal
osteophyte
formation

new bone
formation
anteriorly

anterior
margin of
intervertebral
disc

scalloping
of posterior
aspect of
vertebral bodies

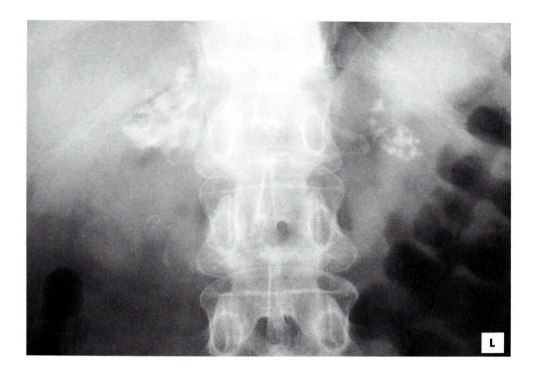

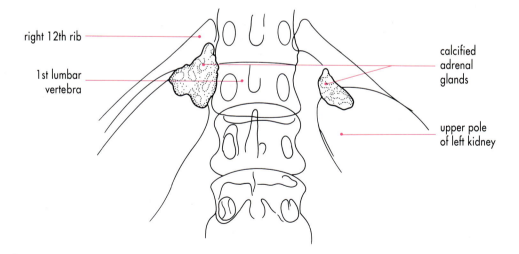

right 12th rib

1st lumbar
vertebra

calcified
adrenal
glands

upper pole
of left kidney

Fig. 1.9 Addison's disease: calcified adrenal glands. This coned anteroposterior (AP) film
of the upper abdomen demonstrates calcified adrenal glands, seen in some patients with Addison's
disease. An identical appearance, however, may be found incidentally in patients without evidence of
adrenal disease (the so-called 'idiopathic' calcification of the adrenals).

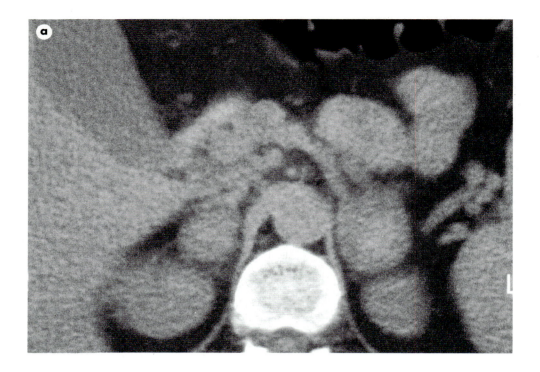

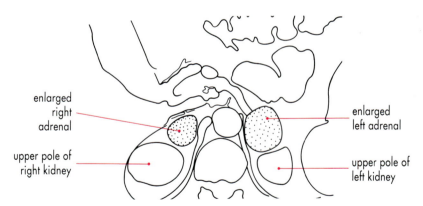

enlarged
right
adrenal

enlarged
left adrenal

upper pole of
right kidney

upper pole of
left kidney

**Fig. 1.10 Addison's disease: enlarged adrenal glands demonstrated by
computed tomography (CT).** The CT scan (a) shows bilateral adrenal enlargement in a patient
taking anticoagulant therapy who presented with the features of acute adrenal insufficiency. The
adrenals show increased density compared with the soft tissues indicating recent haemorrhage. The
follow-up scan seven months later, shows shrinkage of both the right (b) and left (c) adrenal glands,
which have lost their normal contour.

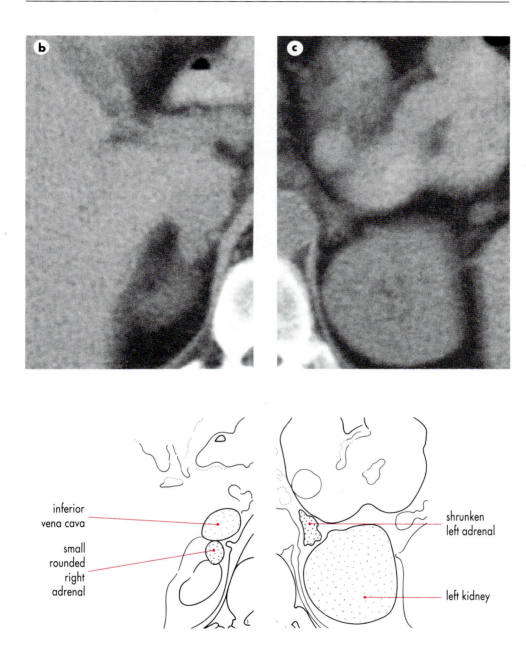

Fig. 1.10

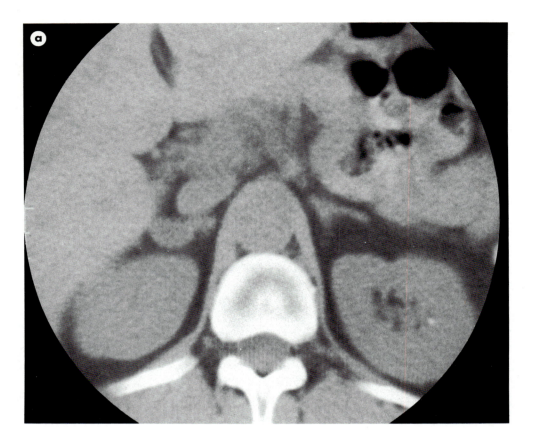

Fig. 1.11

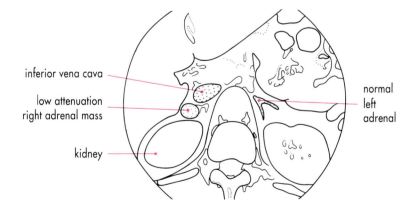

inferior vena cava

low attenuation
right adrenal mass

kidney

normal
left
adrenal

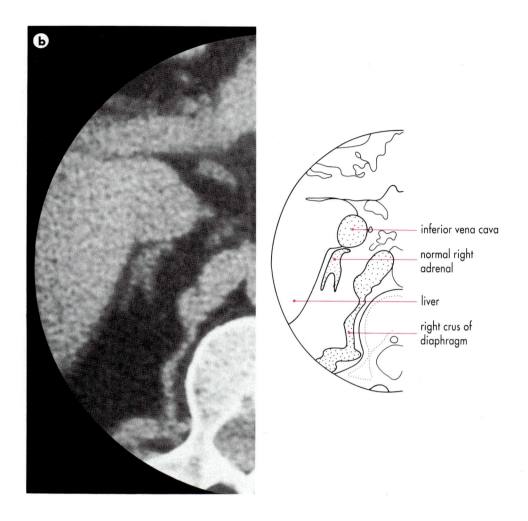

inferior vena cava

normal right
adrenal

liver

right crus of
diaphragm

Fig. 1.11 Conn's syndrome: right adrenal adenoma demonstrated by CT (with normal adrenal glands for comparison). Conn's syndrome is caused by either adrenal hyperplasia or an adrenal tumour, the majority of which are small adenomas. Scan (a) shows a 1cm tumour in the right adrenal gland, lying between the inferior vena cava (IVC) and the right kidney, and a normal left adrenal gland. The tumour is of low attenuation when compared with the soft tissues. This feature is often seen in Conn's tumours. Venous sampling to measure aldosterone levels may be required to confirm the CT findings and may detect tumours too small to be visualised on CT. Significantly elevated aldosterone levels from both adrenal glands usually indicates bilateral hyperplasia. Scan (b) shows a normal right adrenal gland for comparison. The short adrenal body is situated immediately posterior to the IVC. It divides into two parallel limbs which lie between the liver and the right crus of the diaphragm.

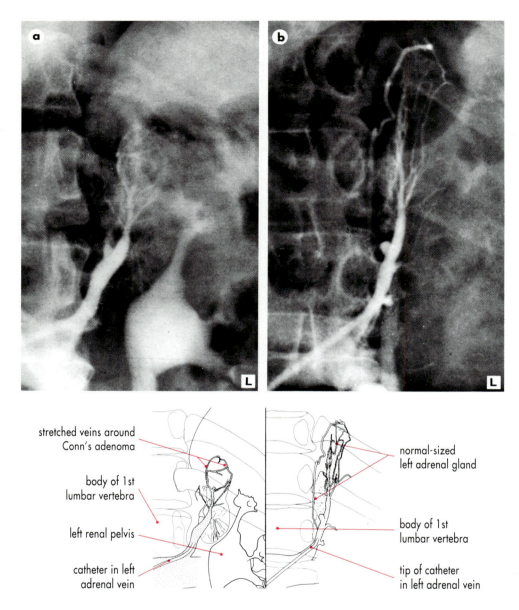

stretched veins around
Conn's adenoma

body of 1st
lumbar vertebra

left renal pelvis

catheter in left
adrenal vein

normal-sized
left adrenal gland

body of 1st
lumbar vertebra

tip of catheter
in left adrenal vein

Fig. 1.12 Conn's adenoma in the left adrenal gland: demonstrated by venography (with normal venogram for comparison). Film (a) shows the typical venographic appearance of a Conn's adenoma. The catheter tip is in the left adrenal vein and contrast medium has filled veins stretched around a 1cm tumour in the superior pole of the adrenal gland. This appearance should be compared with that of a normal left adrenal venogram (b). Blood for aldosterone estimation should be taken from the adrenal vein prior to venography because of the risk of extravasation of contrast medium during that procedure. Even careful venography carries a small risk of adrenal infarction which could result in adrenal insufficiency if both adrenal glands are compromised.

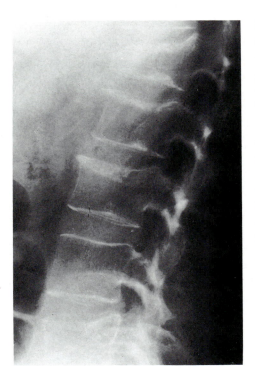

Fig. 1.13 Cushing's syndrome: osteoporosis and vertebral fractures.

Cushing's syndrome, when severe, results in generalised osteoporosis and this lateral film of the lumbar spine shows the typical appearance. The bone density is reduced and the cortical margins of the bones are thin. There is marked collapse of the body of the first lumbar vertebra, with marginal condensation of the superior borders of the bodies of the second and third. In the dorsal spine multiple vertebral fractures may lead to a pronounced kyphosis. It should be noted that the radiological appearances of osteoporosis affecting the spine are similar whatever the cause.

marked collapse of the
body of 1st lumbar
vertebra

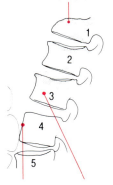

1

2

3

4

5

thin   generalised loss
cortex   of bone density

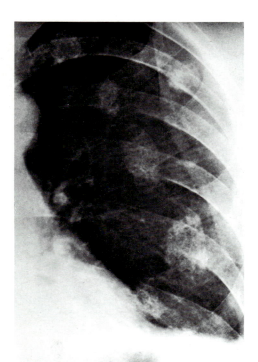

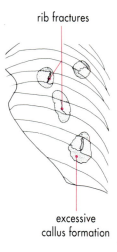

rib fractures

excessive
callus formation

Fig. 1.14 Cushing's syndrome: rib fractures. Spontaneous asymptomatic rib fractures are characteristic of Cushing's syndrome and this coned view shows the typical appearance. Multiple rib fractures are surrounded by excessive callus formation. In some patients, in addition to obvious rib fractures, characteristic widening of the anterior ends of the ribs resulting from numerous stress infractions may be seen.

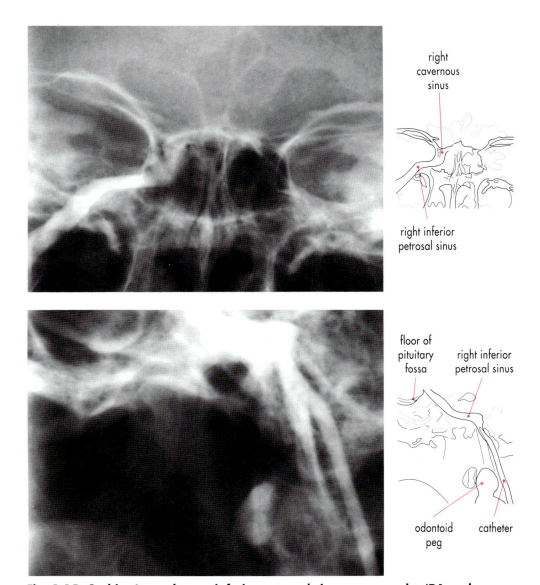

Fig. 1.15 Cushing's syndrome: inferior petrosal sinus venography (PA and lateral) to confirm catheter position prior to venous sampling. Percutaneous catheterisation of one inferior petrosal sinus, or if possible both simultaneously, is useful in the investigation of ACTH-dependent Cushing's syndrome. The finding of a 2:1 gradient in ACTH levels in venous samples from the inferior petrosal sinus(es) compared with peripheral blood suggests that the syndrome is likely to be of pituitary origin but is only seen in 50 per cent of cases. However, if 100µg corticotrophin releasing hormone CRH41 is given intravenously, a rise in ACTH levels in the petrosal sinuses of over twice the basal value establishes a diagnosis of pituitary dependent Cushing's disease in 80 per cent of cases and may lateralise a microadenoma to one side of the fossa. Venous sampling from other sites may help to locate an ectopic source of ACTH production.

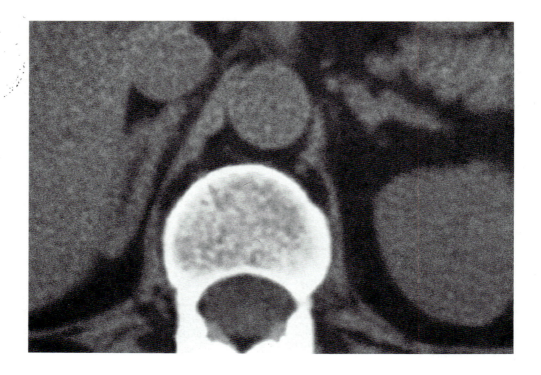

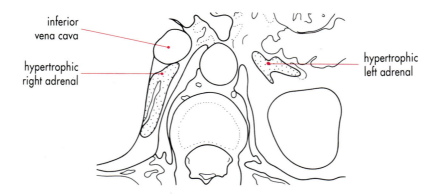

inferior
vena cava

hypertrophic
right adrenal

hypertrophic
left adrenal

Fig. 1.16 Cushing's syndrome: hypertrophy of the adrenal glands demonstrated by CT. Most cases of Cushing's syndrome are caused by increased ACTH production by the pituitary gland. The remainder are due either to an ectopic ACTH-producing tumour or to a primary adrenal tumour (adenoma or carcinoma). Increasing ACTH levels result in adrenal hyperplasia with accompanying hypertrophy. Small changes in size cannot be detected by CT and the adrenals may therefore appear normal. More marked hypertrophy can be shown as thickening of the limbs of the gland with convexity of the margins. The normal configuration is, however, retained. (Compare with the CT appearance of normal adrenals Fig. 1.11.)

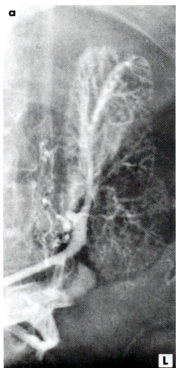
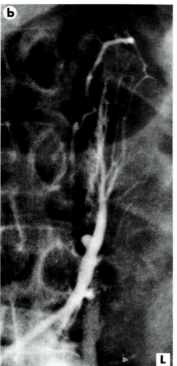
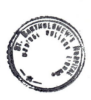

**Fig. 1.17
Cushing's
syndrome:
hypertrophied left
adrenal gland
demonstrated by
venography (with
normal venogram
for comparison).**

Film (a) was obtained
prior to venous
sampling and shows
the venographic
appearances of one of
a pair of hypertrophied
adrenal glands. The tip
of the catheter is in the
left adrenal vein and
contrast medium has
filled small veins within
the enlarged gland.
A segment of the left
renal vein has been
partially outlined. The
appearances should be
compared with those of
a normal-sized left
adrenal gland (b).

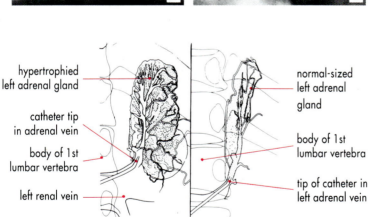
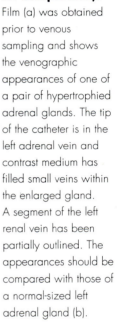

hypertrophied
left adrenal gland

catheter tip
in adrenal vein

body of 1st
lumbar vertebra

left renal vein

normal-sized
left adrenal
gland

body of 1st
lumbar vertebra

tip of catheter in
left adrenal vein

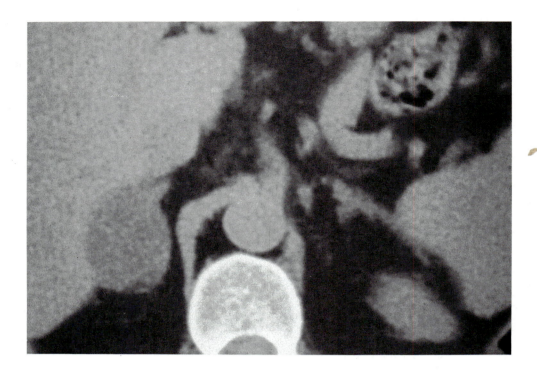

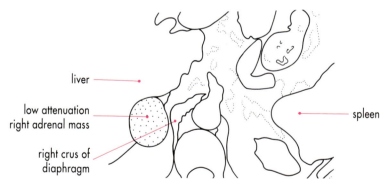

liver
low attenuation
right adrenal mass
right crus of
diaphragm
spleen

Fig. 1.18 Cushing's syndrome: right adrenal adenoma demonstrated by CT.
Adrenal adenomas causing Cushing's syndrome are usually 2–5cm in size. They are readily detected by CT because of the contrast provided by the abundant retroperitoneal fat which is present in most patients. This scan shows a 3.5cm rounded mass in the right adrenal gland. It lies immediately behind the IVC and between the liver and the right crus of the diaphragm.

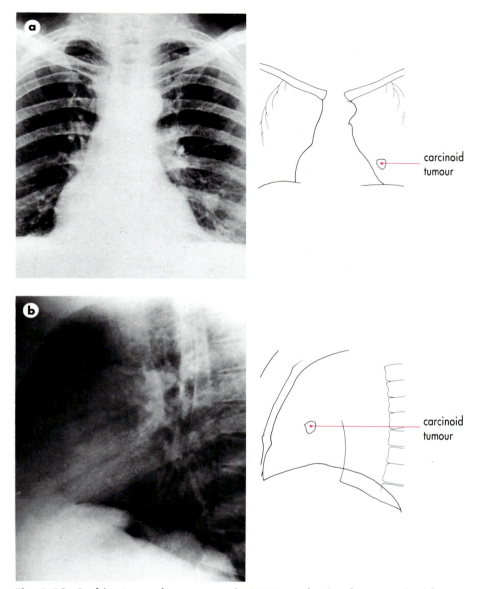

Fig. 1.19 Cushing's syndrome: ectopic ACTH production by a carcinoid tumour of the lung. Cushing's syndrome sometimes results from ectopic ACTH production by tumours, particularly of the lung, thymus or pancreas. Such tumours may be very difficult to locate. Although a few may be detected by conventional radiographic techniques, others require CT scanning or venous sampling for their identification, and some are never found. The PA chest film (a) shows a small mass in the left lower zone. There is some generalised loss of bone density and the patient appears fat. On the lateral view (b) the mass is shown to lie in the lingular segment of the left upper lobe. The patient had Cushing's syndrome secondary to ectopic ACTH production by a benign bronchial carcinoid tumour of the lung.

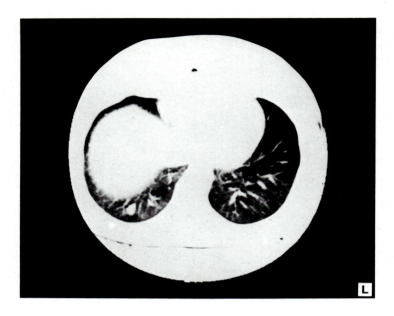

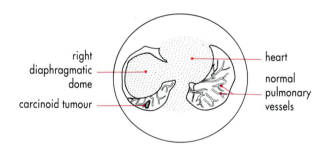

right
diaphragmatic
dome

heart

normal
pulmonary
vessels

carcinoid tumour

Fig. 1.20 Cushing's syndrome: ACTH-secreting carcinoid tumour of the lung demonstrated by CT. The 7mm nodule in the right costophrenic recess represents a small malignant carcinoid tumour secreting ACTH. It could not be seen on either chest radiography or conventional tomography. Removal of the tumour cured the patient. (Reproduced by courtesy of the British Medical Journal).

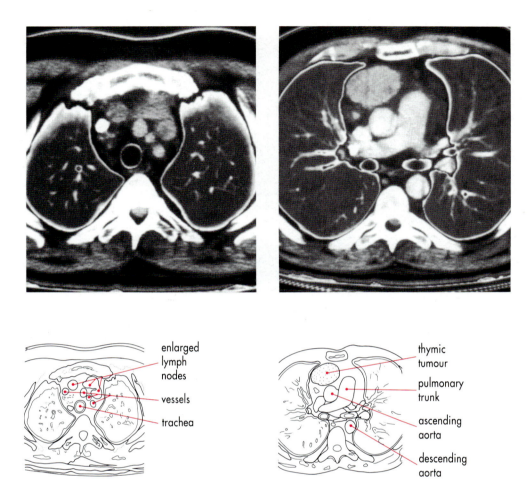

Fig. 1.21 Cushing's syndrome: malignant thymic ACTH-secreting carcinoid tumour demonstrated by CT. Ectopic ACTH can be produced by carcinoid tumours of the thymus. These enhanced CT scans show in the right picture a 4cm ACTH-producing tumour lying just in front of the ascending aorta. The tumour has enhanced slightly with contrast medium but not as markedly as the vascular structures. The left scan shows enlarged anterior mediastinal lymph nodes at a higher level.

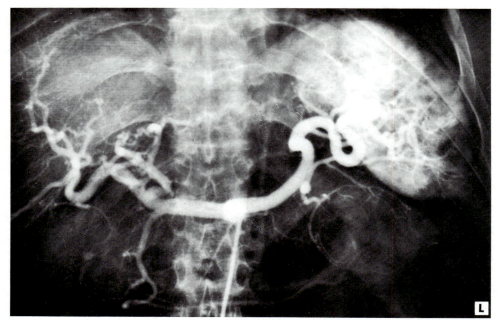

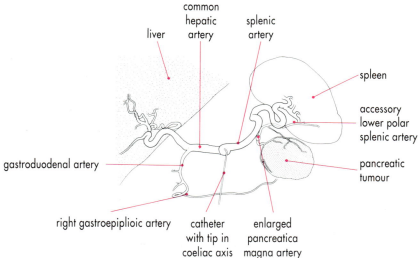

liver

common
hepatic
artery

splenic
artery

spleen

accessory
lower polar
splenic artery

gastroduodenal artery

pancreatic
tumour

right gastroepiploic artery

catheter
with tip in
coeliac axis

enlarged
pancreatica
magna artery

Fig. 1.22 Cushing's syndrome: ectopic ACTH production by an islet cell tumour of the pancreas demonstrated by angiography. This picture shows the arterial phase of a coeliac axis arteriogram. The procedure was carried out to define the blood supply of a pancreatic tumour which had been previously demonstrated by CT. The pancreatica magna artery is enlarged and its branches are stretched over the surface of a large pancreatic tumour. The splenic vein was shown to be patent on later films. At operation a large tumour of the pancreas was removed. Histological examination showed an islet cell tumour which was thought to be malignant. The tumour contained ACTH and the patient was cured of his Cushing's syndrome upon its removal.

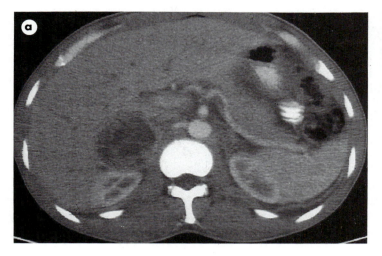

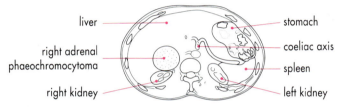

liver — stomach
right adrenal phaeochromocytoma — coeliac axis
right kidney — spleen
— left kidney

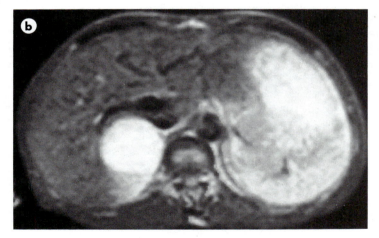

liver — stomach
right adrenal phaeochromocytoma — spleen

Fig. 1.23 Adrenal phaeochromocytoma: right adrenal tumour demonstrated by CT and MRI. Most adrenal phaeochromocytomas can be detected by CT because they are usually 3cm or more in size. The enhanced CT scan (a) shows an inhomogeneous, predominantly low density 5cm mass replacing the right adrenal gland. Small tumours may show uniform contrast enhancement. Larger tumours often show areas of low density due to tumour necrosis, as in this case. Magnetic resonance imaging (MRI) can also demonstrate adrenal masses well. Phaeochromocytomas show most clearly on MRI in the T2-weighted images as a mass with a high signal, as in scan (b).

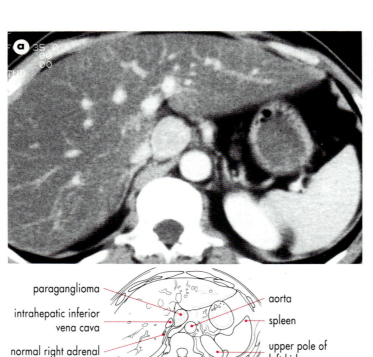

paraganglioma — aorta

intrahepatic inferior
vena cava — spleen

normal right adrenal — upper pole of
left kidney

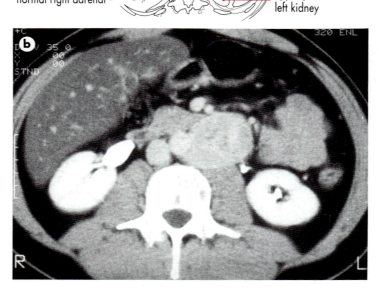

fatty liver

aorta — para-aortic
paraganglioma

extrarenal pelvis
of right kidney — left kidney

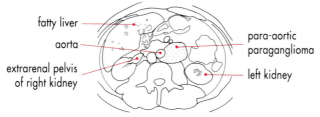

Fig. 1.24
Para-aortic
paragangliomas
demonstrated by
CT. If an adrenal tumour
is not shown on CT in a
patient with strong
clinical evidence of a
phaeochromocytoma, it is
likely that the tumour lies
at an ectopic site along
the sympathetic chain.
The majority of such
paragangliomas occur in
the para-aortic region or
around the renal hilum,
and may be visible on
CT. Scan (a) shows a
small tumour lying anterior
to and separate from the
right adrenal. A second
larger tumour is present to
the left of the aorta at the
level of the kidneys (b).
Both were confirmed as
benign paragangliomas
at surgery. To detect
tumours at other ectopic
sites or those too small
to be seen on CT, [123]I
metaiodobenzylguanidine
(MIBG) radionuclide
scanning (see Chapter 3
Figs. 3.16 & 3.19) or
venous sampling for
catecholamine levels is
required.

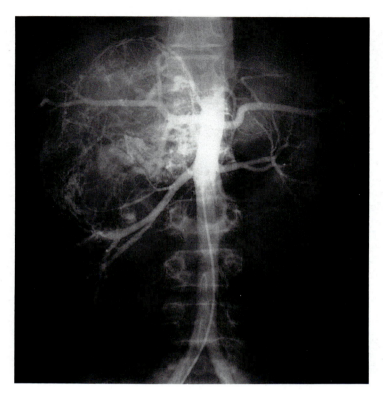

Fig. 1.25 Adrenal phaeochromocytoma: large vascular tumour demonstrated by arteriography.

Arteriography has now been largely superseded by CT, MIBG scanning and venous sampling for the detection of phaeochromocytomas. The procedure is hazardous unless adequate medical α- and β-adrenergic blockade has been given and should be undertaken only if really essential. In this patient angiography was carried out to determine the arterial supply and venous drainage of the known tumour prior to surgery. Arteriography still has a place in identifying an ectopic phaeochromocytoma when its approximate location has been shown by venous sampling or MIBG scanning, and CT examination is negative.

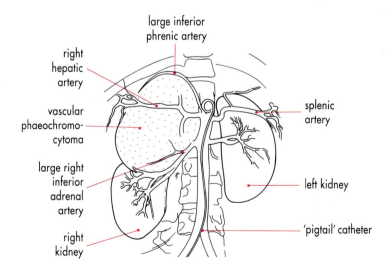

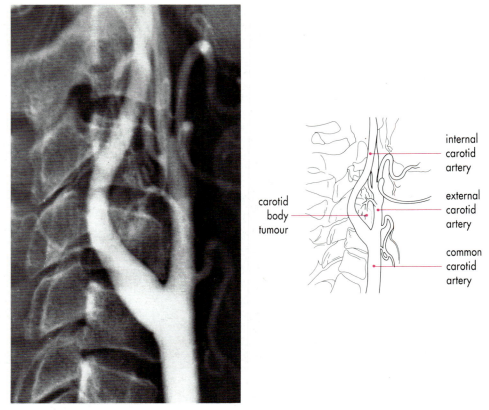

Fig. 1.26 Carotid body tumour: demonstration by angiography. This patient with persistent hypertension after the removal of a left adrenal phaeochromocytoma had elevated levels of catecholamines in the right side of the neck on venous sampling. Subsequent carotid arteriography demonstrated a typical carotid body tumour. On this lateral film the carotid bifurcation is seen to be splayed by the tumour which lies between the origins of the internal and external carotid arteries. The blood supply of the tumour arises from the proximal external carotid artery and a tumour blush is present.

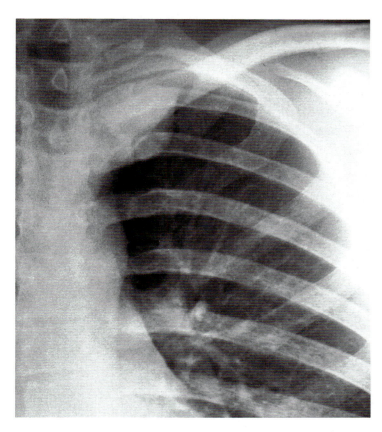

Fig. 1.27 Malignant paraganglioma in the left upper chest. This coned view shows a mass with a well-defined margin lying in the left upper paravertebral region. The patient complained of occasional headaches and sweating but was normotensive. At operation, however, the blood pressure rose steeply while the tumour was being handled. Histological examination showed a paraganglioma which was originally thought to be benign. Seven years later, however, the tumour recurred in the chest and metastatic paraganglioma was found on biopsy of a skull lesion. The patient is still alive, seventeen years after initial presentation.

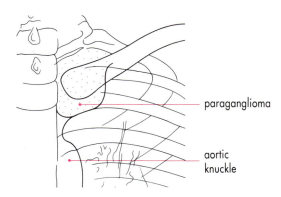

paraganglioma

aortic knuckle

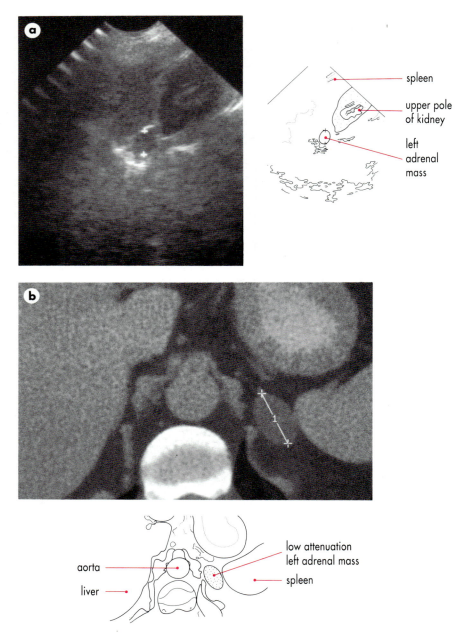

Fig. 1.28 Nonfunctional left adrenal tumour: ultrasound and CT scans. This 2cm mass was an incidental finding on ultrasonography (a). CT (b) confirmed that the mass was of adrenal origin and also showed that it had a relatively low attenuation suggestive of adrenocortical origin. In this situation, a biochemical screen is indicated to determine whether or not there is evidence of endocrine disease. If this is normal a follow-up scan should be done to exclude an increase in size, indicative of malignancy. Nonfunctional adrenal masses are quite frequently found on CT and surgery is unwarranted in most cases.

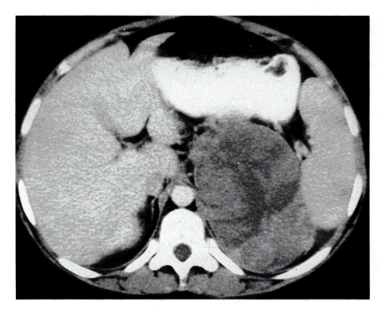

Fig. 1.29 Adrenal carcinoma: CT scan. This 10cm left adrenal mass shows the characteristic CT appearances of an adrenal carcinoma. Adrenal carcinomas usually measure 6cm or more at the time of presentation and show inhomogeneous enhancement following the injection of intravenous contrast medium. Enlarged lymph nodes or metastatic spread elsewhere may also be shown. This patient had a pulmonary metastasis on chest X-ray.

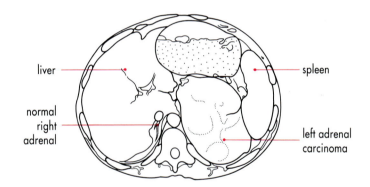

liver

spleen

normal right adrenal

left adrenal carcinoma

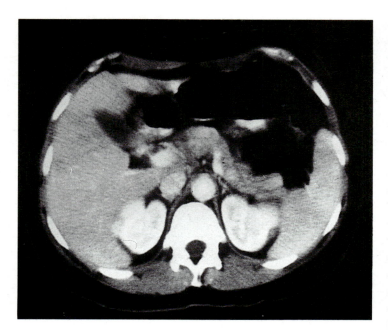

**Fig. 1.30
Insulinoma:
demonstrated by
contrast-enhanced
CT.** These islet cell
tumours of the pancreas
are often less than
1.5 cm in diameter, are
multiple in 10 per cent
of cases and are
occasionally malignant.
Their demonstration by
CT requires a meticulous
technique, using thin
contiguous sections
and rapid sequence
scanning after a bolus
of contrast medium.
Even small insulinomas
can be detected by CT
because of their intense
enhancement, as seen
in this scan.

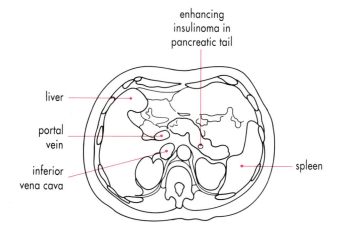

enhancing
insulinoma in
pancreatic tail

liver

portal
vein

inferior
vena cava

spleen

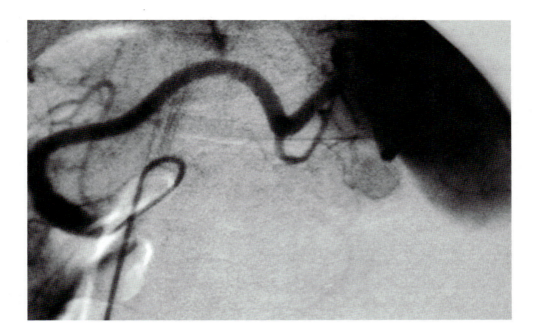

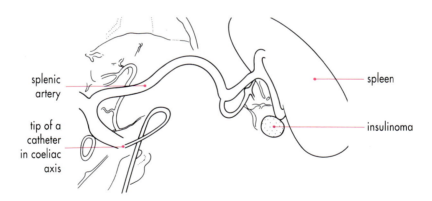

splenic artery

tip of a catheter in coeliac axis

spleen

insulinoma

Fig. 1.31 Insulinoma: demonstrated by intra-arterial digital subtraction angiography (DSA). Selective or superselective arterial catheterisation is required together with gas distension of the stomach and paralysis of the bowel. Multiple projections may be necessary, as in this patient where the small insulinoma in the tail of the pancreas (confirmed surgically) was only clearly shown on DSA films obtained in the 45° left anterior oblique projection. Angiography may produce a false positive 'blush' from the gut or splenunculus and this problem can be resolved by combining angiography with CT, which will show whether the 'blush' is truly pancreatic (see Fig. 1.32).

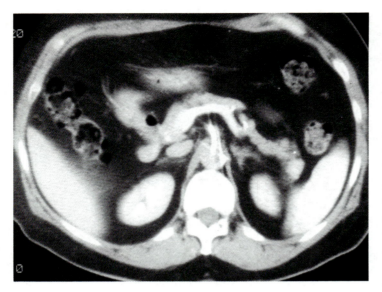

Fig. 1.32
Insulinoma:
demonstrated by
CT angiography.
CT angiography is
probably the most
sensitive means of
detecting small islet cell
tumours pre-operatively.
This CT scan was
obtained immediately
after the injection of
contrast medium into
the coeliac axis.
It shows a small
insulinoma in the tail of
the pancreas, lying at
the splenic hilum,
which was not
detected on the initial
angiogram.
Transhepatic venous
sampling may be
helpful in locating an
insulinoma not detected
by CT and/or
angiography.

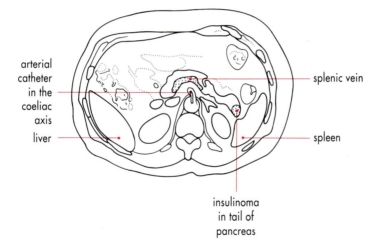

arterial
catheter
in the
coeliac
axis

liver

splenic vein

spleen

insulinoma
in tail of
pancreas

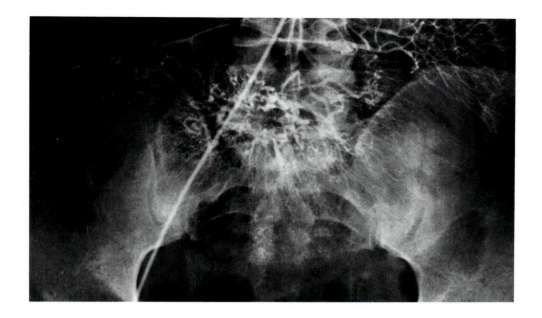

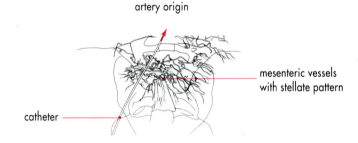

to superior mesenteric
artery origin

mesenteric vessels
with stellate pattern

catheter

Fig. 1.33 Carcinoid tumour: characteristic angiographic appearance of mesenteric involvement. This film from the arterial phase of a superior mesenteric arteriogram demonstrates the typical angiographic appearance of a carcinoid tumour which has invaded the mesentery. Invasion results in thickening and foreshortening of the mesentery. The arteries become very tortuous and are drawn into a characteristic stellate pattern. Arterial narrowing distal to the tumour frequently occurs.

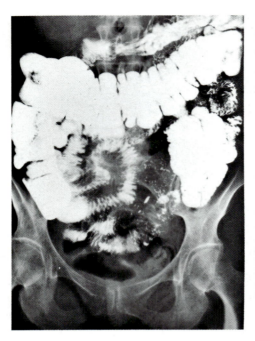

Fig. 1.34 Carcinoid tumour: distal ileal involvement. This 80 minute follow-through film shows an abnormal distal ileum with mesenteric thickening, nodular masses invading the bowel wall and angulation and tethering of mucosal folds. These appearances are characteristic of carcinoid tumour and reflect invasion by the tumour with an extensive fibroblastic response. Metastatic carcinoma to the mesentery can cause a similar appearance.

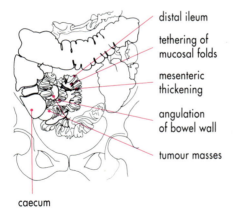

distal ileum

tethering of
mucosal folds

mesenteric
thickening

angulation
of bowel wall

tumour masses

caecum

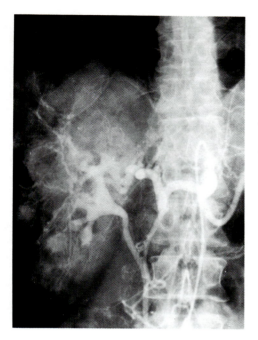

Fig. 1.35 Carcinoid tumour: hypervascular hepatic metastases.
Hepatic metastases from a carcinoid tumour are characteristically hypervascular and this film of the arterial phase of a coeliac axis arteriogram shows multiple tumour blushes throughout the liver.
A similar appearance is produced by other hypervascular hepatic metastases such as those from a renal cell carcinoma.

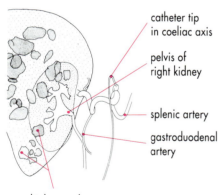

catheter tip
in coeliac axis

pelvis of
right kidney

splenic artery

gastroduodenal
artery

multiple vascular
metastases in liver
from carcinoid tumour

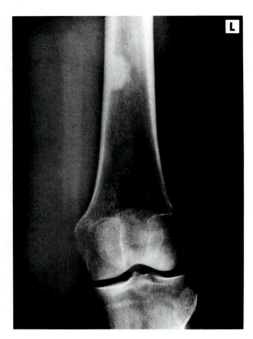

Fig. 1.36 Carcinoid tumour: sclerotic bony metastasis. Bony metastases from malignant carcinoid tumours are characteristically densely sclerotic. This AP film of the distal femur and knee shows the typical appearance of such an intramedullary lesion. The primary tumour was in the rectum. (Carcinoid tumour: ectopic ACTH production. See under Cushing's syndrome Figs. 1.19–1.21.)

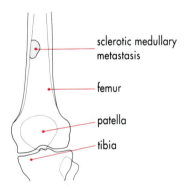

sclerotic medullary metastasis

femur

patella

tibia

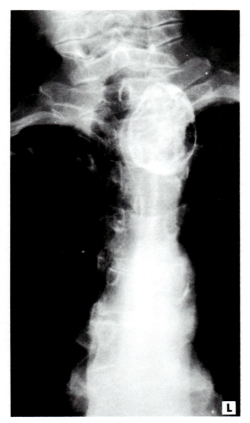

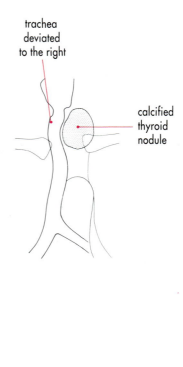

trachea
deviated
to the right

calcified
thyroid
nodule

Fig. 1.37 Goitre: calcified thyroid nodule. This AP film of the thoracic inlet shows the typical appearance of a large calcified thyroid nodule which is slightly displacing the trachea to the right side. Most goitres, however, do not show calcification. Calcified goitres are usually benign but may be malignant.

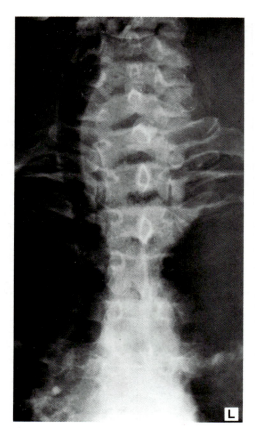

Fig. 1.38 Goitre: deviation and narrowing of the trachea. This AP view of the thoracic inlet shows marked displacement of the trachea to the right by a large left-sided goitre which extends inferiorly to just below the sternal notch. The trachea is slightly narrowed in its transverse diameter just above the level of the thoracic inlet. No calcification can be seen within the goitre. Although any displacement or narrowing of the trachea in the AP plane can be readily assessed on a lateral view of the thoracic inlet, it may be difficult to determine whether or not there is any significant extension of a cervical goitre into the mediastinum.

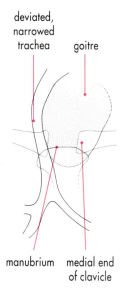

deviated, narrowed trachea   goitre

manubrium   medial end of clavicle

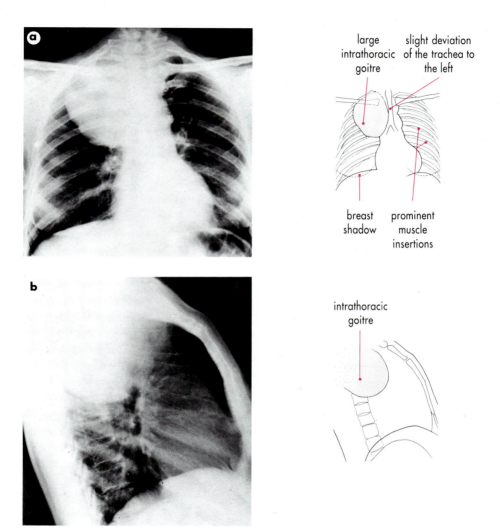

Fig. 1.39 Intrathoracic goitre in acromegaly. The PA chest film (a) shows a large mass in the right upper chest which is confluent with the mediastinum medially and has a well-defined lateral margin. The mass does not contain any obvious calcification and is only slightly displacing the trachea to the left. The right lateral view (b) shows a clearly defined mass lying posteriorly. The patient had presented with a goitre and had noticed some enlargement of the hands and feet. There were no symptoms of dysphagia or of thyrotoxicosis. The mass in the chest was subsequently shown on radionuclide and CT scans to be in continuity with the cervical goitre. The patient was also found to have a pituitary tumour and acromegaly. Prominent muscle insertions can be seen on the PA chest film at the lower borders of the ribs but no bony changes of acromegaly are present in the dorsal spine (see Fig. 1.7). At the combined surgical approach of cervical incision and a right posterolateral thoractomy, the large mass in the right side of the mediastinum was confirmed to be continuous with an enlarged right lobe of the thyroid gland and was removed. Histological examination showed that the mass was a large colloid goitre.

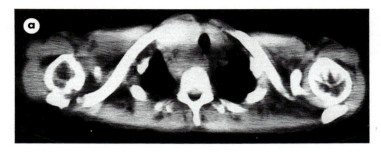

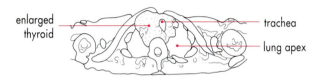

enlarged
thyroid — trachea

— lung apex

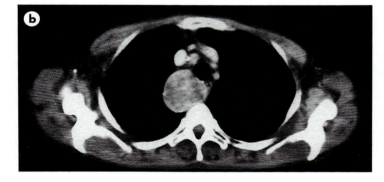

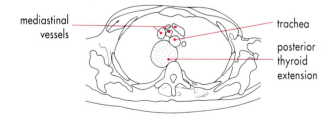

mediastinal
vessels — trachea

— posterior
thyroid
extension

**Fig. 1.40
Intrathoracic
goitre: CT scans.**
These are of a different
patient to Fig. 1.39.
The higher scan (a)
shows bilateral thyroid
enlargement with
narrowing and
displacement of the
trachea. The density of
thyroid tissue on
unenhanced CT is usually
higher than that of other
soft tissues because of
the iodine content of the
gland. This is not
particularly obvious in
this patient. The lower
scan (b) shows
extension of the right
lobe into the posterior
mediastinum with
patchy enhancement
following intravenous
contrast.

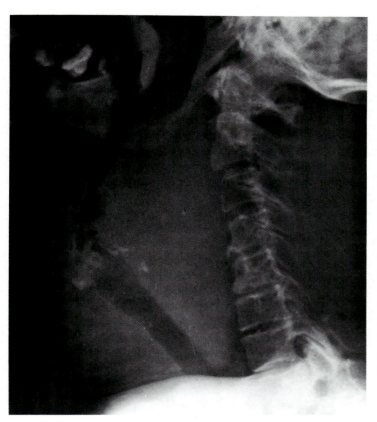

Fig. 1.41 Carcinoma of the thyroid: retrotracheal extension of tumour. This lateral view of the neck shows massive soft tissue swelling with marked anterior displacement of the trachea which is compressed in its anteroposterior diameter. The displacement is due to gross retrotracheal extension of the thyroid and is indicative of malignancy. This patient had an anaplastic carcinoma of the thyroid.

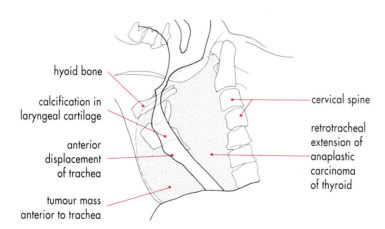

hyoid bone

calcification in laryngeal cartilage

anterior displacement of trachea

tumour mass anterior to trachea

cervical spine

retrotracheal extension of anaplastic carcinoma of thyroid

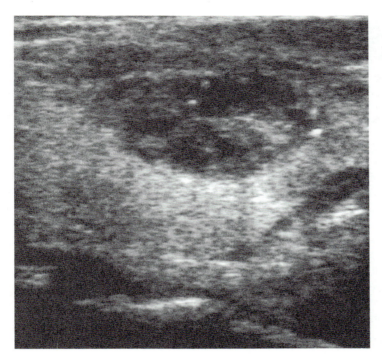

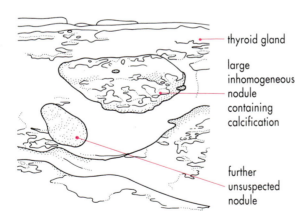

thyroid gland

large
inhomogeneous
nodule
containing
calcification

further
unsuspected
nodule

**Fig. 1.42
Multinodular
goitre: ultrasound
scan.** This longitudinal
scan shows a large
nodule containing
specks of calcium
which was 'cold' on
radionuclide scanning
(see Chapter 3
Fig. 3.6). Ultrasound
revealed further nodules,
consistent with a
multinodular goitre.
Fine needle aspiration
confirmed the benign
nature of the 'cold'
nodule. In patients who
appear to have a
solitary thyroid nodule
clinically, which is
'cold' on radionuclide
scanning, neck
ultrasound can be of
value. It will show if the
nodule is cystic or
solid. Solitary solid
thyroid lesions need
further investigation
because they may be
malignant. The
presence of unsuspected
further nodules,
however, usually
indicates a multinodular
goitre.

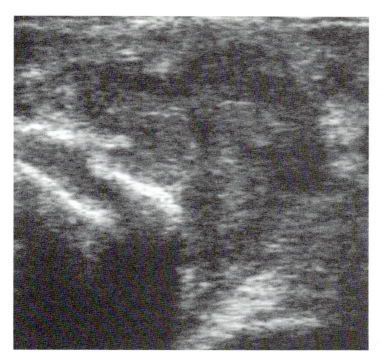

Fig. 1.43 Thyroid carcinoma: ultrasound scan. This transverse scan shows an irregular, hypoechoic mass in the left lobe of the thyroid in a patient with metastatic disease but no known primary. Ultrasound-guided fine needle aspiration yielded abnormal cells consistent with an anaplastic carcinoma.

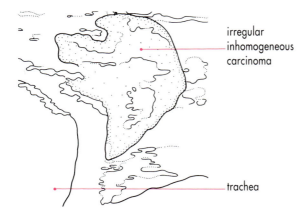

irregular
inhomogeneous
carcinoma

trachea

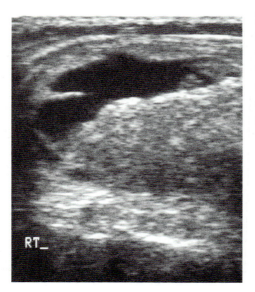

Fig. 1.44 Hürthle cell tumour: ultrasound scan. This transverse scan shows an unusual partly cystic mass in the right lobe of the thyroid in a patient with gradual thyroid enlargement over two years. Fine needle aspiration showed large numbers of Hürthle cells and surgery confirmed a Hürthle cell tumour.

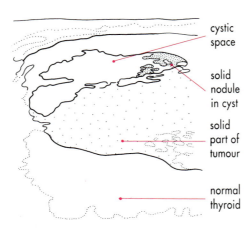

cystic space

solid nodule in cyst

solid part of tumour

normal thyroid

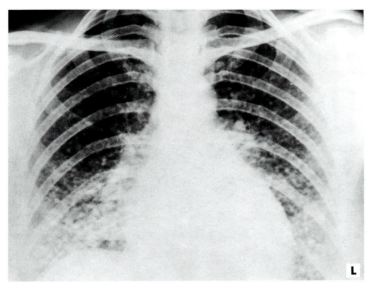

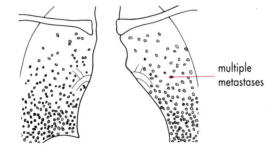

multiple metastases

Fig. 1.45
Carcinoma of the thyroid: 'snow storm' appearance of pulmonary metastases. This PA chest film shows multiple small nodular opacities throughout both lungs, most marked at the bases, the characteristic 'snow storm' appearance of pulmonary metastases from carcinoma of the thyroid. Such metastatic deposits may remain unchanged over a long period of time due to a very low grade of malignancy and may take up and be treated with [131]I.

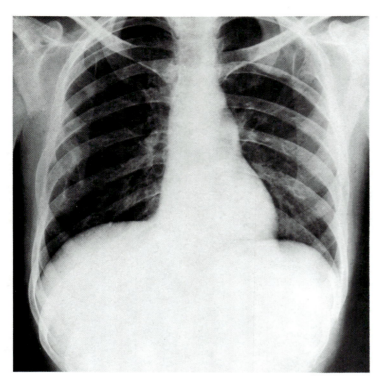

**Fig. 1.46
Carcinoma of the
thyroid: chest
radiograph
showing expanded
bony metastases.**
This PA chest film shows
multiple osteolytic bony
metastases. Those
involving the right
scapula and the left
fourth and ninth ribs
show marked expansion
of bone. Carcinoma
of the thyroid
characteristically gives
rise to osteolytic
metastases, sometimes
accompanied by
marked expansion of
bone, as in this patient.
The appearance is,
however, not diagnostic
because metastatic
renal cell carcinoma,
multiple myeloma, and
occasionally metastatic
carcinoma of the breast
may also cause
similar bone expansion.
Such thyroid carcinoma
metastases may, but
do not necessarily,
show up on routine
radionuclide bone
scanning.

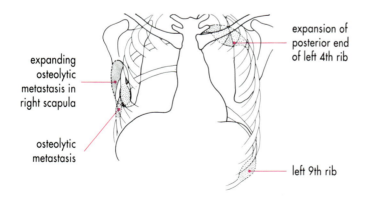

expanding
osteolytic
metastasis in
right scapula

osteolytic
metastasis

expansion of
posterior end
of left 4th rib

left 9th rib

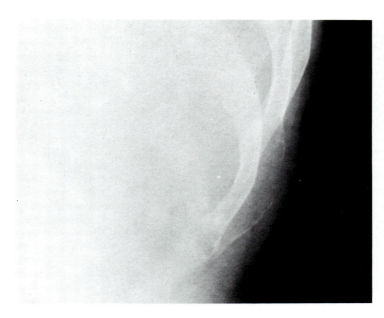

**Fig. 1.47
Carcinoma of the
thyroid: close-up
view of an
expanded rib
metastasis.** This
coned view of the left
ninth rib of the same
patient as in Fig. 1.46
clearly shows the
medullary destruction
and expansion with
thinning of the
overlying cortex.

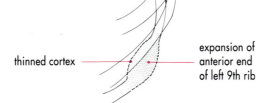

thinned cortex ——————— expansion of
anterior end
of left 9th rib

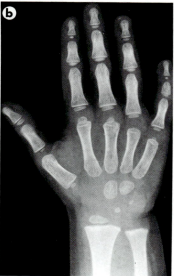
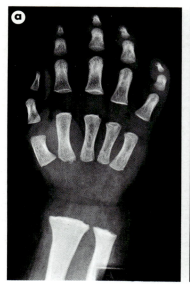

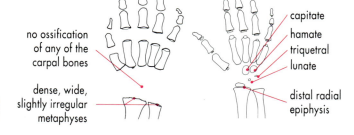

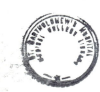

no ossification
of any of the
carpal bones

dense, wide,
slightly irregular
metaphyses

capitate
hamate
triquetral
lunate

distal radial
epiphysis

Fig. 1.48 Hypothyroidism in childhood: delay in skeletal maturation (with normal hand for comparison). This PA film (a) of the hand of a three-year-old hypothyroid boy demonstrates the characteristic retardation of skeletal growth. The bones of the hand are smaller than normal reflecting the generalised delay in growth that occurs and ossification has not yet started in any of the carpal bones or secondary epiphyses. Irregularity and increased density of the metaphyses occurs and, in this view, these changes are best seen in the distal radius and ulna. The appearances should be compared with those of the hand of a normal boy of similar age (b).

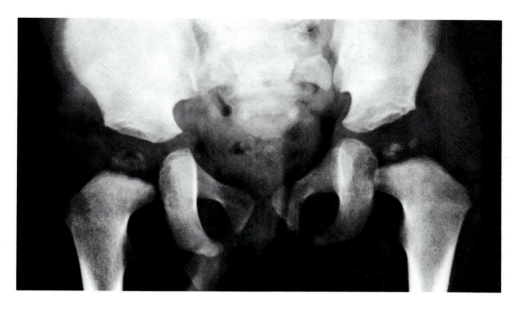

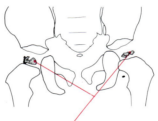

fragmented proximal
femoral secondary
epiphyses

Fig. 1.49 Hypothyroidism in childhood: fragmentation of the femoral capital epiphyses. This AP view of the pelvis shows delay in ossification, with fragmentation and hypoplasia of the femoral capital epiphyses. Fragmentation of the ossification centres of the femoral heads might suggest the diagnosis of bilateral Perthes' disease; however, symmetrical involvement would be excessively rare in that condition.

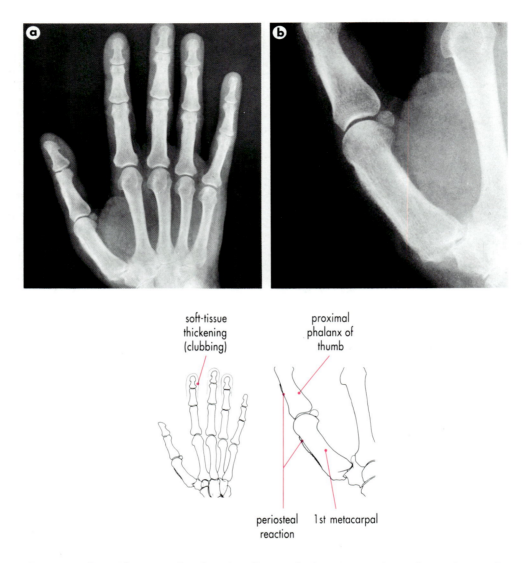

Fig. 1.50 Thyroid acropachy: hand radiograph showing periosteal reaction and clubbing. Thyroid acropachy occurs as part of Graves' disease and consists of clubbing of the fingers and toes, usually associated with exophthalmos and pretibial myxoedema. Bone changes are not necessarily part of the syndrome although they are frequently present. The PA film (a) of a hand shows the characteristic periosteal reaction of thyroid acropachy along the radial aspect of the shaft of the first metacarpal, the typical site. Soft tissue thickening is evident around some of the distal phalanges. The coned view (b) of the thumb and first metacarpal better demonstrates the characteristic lace-like appearance of the periosteal reaction. Besides the typical involvement of the first metacarpal, periosteal new bone formation may also occur along the shafts of other metacarpals and the proximal phalanges. In this patient a slight periosteal reaction is also present along the shaft of the proximal phalanx of the thumb.

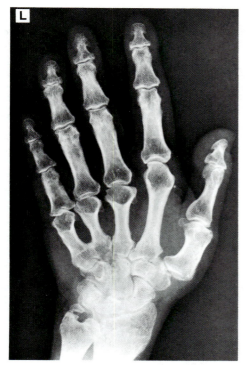

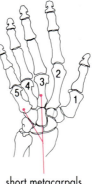

short metacarpals

Fig. 1.51 Pseudohypoparathyroidism: short metacarpals. This PA view of the hand shows short, rather broad metacarpals, an appearance seen in pseudohypoparathyroidism. In this patient, all the metacarpals except the second are rather short but the number involved may be variable.

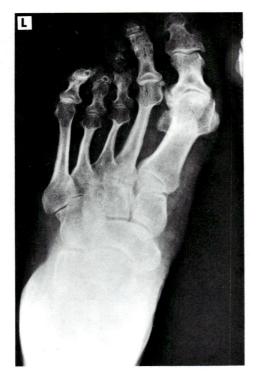

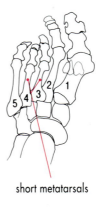

short metatarsals

Fig. 1.52 Pseudohypoparathyroidism: short metatarsals. This AP view of the foot shows a similar appearance to that of the hand, with shortening of the third and fourth metatarsals.

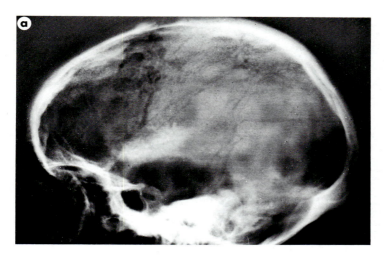

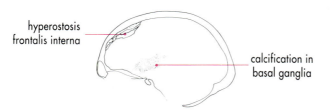

hyperostosis
frontalis interna

calcification in
basal ganglia

**Fig. 1.53
Pseudohypo-
parathyroidism:
calcification in the
basal ganglia.** In
pseudohypoparathy-
roidism, heterotopic
deposits of calcium
phosphate occur in the
soft tissues and most
commonly affect the
basal ganglia. The
lateral (a) and PA (b)
skull films show
characteristic
symmetrical punctate
calcification in the
basal ganglia. Similar
calcification, however,
also occurs in
hypoparathyroidism.
In this patient, slight
hyperostosis frontalis
interna is also present.

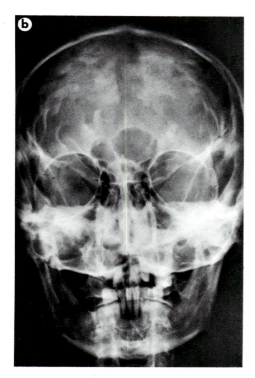

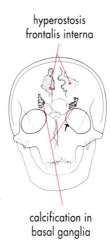

hyperostosis
frontalis interna

calcification in
basal ganglia

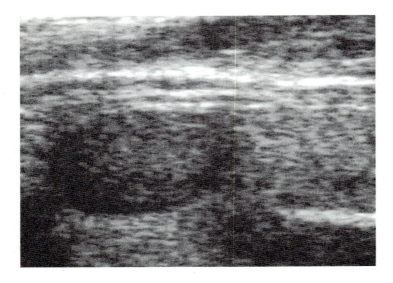

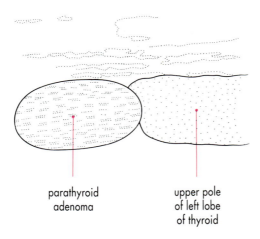

parathyroid
adenoma

upper pole
of left lobe
of thyroid

Fig. 1.54 Parathyroid adenoma: ultrasound scan. The vast majority of parathyroid
adenomas are found on exploration of the neck, providing that the surgeon is experienced.
Pre-operative ultrasonography can, however, be helpful, as in this patient where an enlarged
parathyroid was demonstrated adjacent to the upper pole of the left lobe of the thyroid. The finding of
a solitary enlarged parathyroid gland is likely to indicate an adenoma rather than parathyroid
hyperplasia and is an aid to planning surgery. Intrathyroid parathyroid glands cannot be distinguished
on ultrasonography from other thyroid nodules. (See also Chapter 3 Fig. 3.11.)

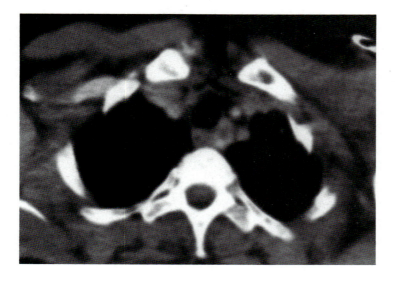

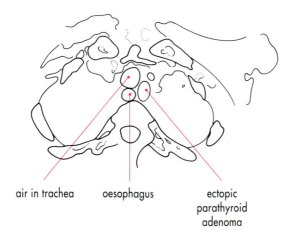

air in trachea   oesophagus   ectopic
                                parathyroid
                                adenoma

Fig. 1.55 Mediastinal parathyroid adenoma: CT scan. CT can be used to try to locate a parathyroid adenoma when neck exploration has failed to identify either a tumour or hyperplasia, or if hypercalcaemia recurs after surgery. This CT scan shows an ectopic parathyroid adenoma lying immediately to the left of the oesophagus. There is rim enhancement following the injection of intravenous contrast medium.

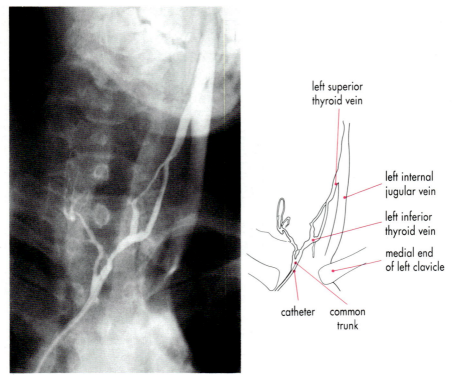

left superior
thyroid vein

left internal
jugular vein

left inferior
thyroid vein

medial end
of left clavicle

catheter   common
trunk

Fig. 1.56 Venous sampling for parathyroid hormone: inferior thyroid venogram. Venous sampling can be undertaken if CT has failed to locate an ectopic tumour. Samples should be taken from mediastinal as well as from thyroid veins. The right and left inferior thyroid veins may join to form a common trunk, as in this patient. The venous anatomy and pattern of drainage may have been altered by previous surgery and not all ectopic tumours will be located by this technique.

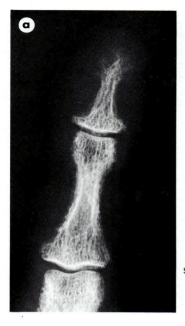

resorption of
tip of distal
phalanx

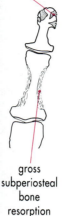

gross
subperiosteal
bone
resorption

Fig. 1.57 Primary hyperparathyroidism: phalanges showing gross subperiosteal bone resorption (with appearance after healing for comparison). Bony changes are now evident radiologically in a minority of patients with primary hyperparathyroidism. Subperiosteal bone resorption is the earliest radiological sign and is specific for hyperparathyroidism. Generalised skeletal demineralisation is a late finding. The film (a) of the middle and distal phalanges of the index finger shows gross subperiosteal bone resorption of the shafts of the phalanges and also of the tip of the distal phalanx. The bone density is decreased and the texture of the cortex shows a 'basket-work' pattern with loss of definition of the normal corticomedullary junction. These appearances of gross hyperparathyroidism should be compared with those in (b) where healing had occurred following removal of a parathyroid adenoma. Although subperiosteal bone resorption classically involves the phalanges, it may also occur at many other sites. These include the outer ends and under-surface of the clavicles, the metaphyseal regions of the growing ends of the long bones, the ischial tuberosities, the pubic bones at the symphysis, the sacroiliac joints and the inner wall of the dorsum sellae.

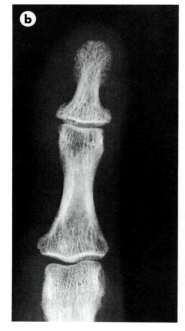

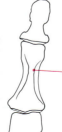

well-defined
corticomedullary
differentiation

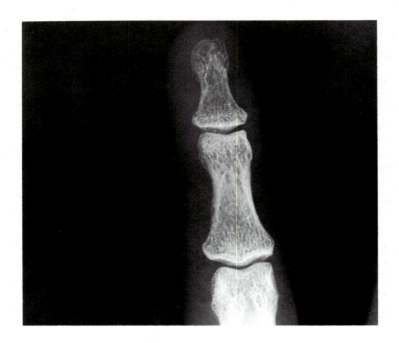

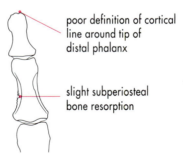

poor definition of cortical
line around tip of
distal phalanx

slight subperiosteal
bone resorption

**Fig. 1.58 Primary hyperparathyroidism: magnification film of the index finger
showing early subperiosteal bone resorption.** This magnified film of the middle and
distal phalanges of the index finger shows the early bony changes of hyperparathyroidism. Slight
subperiosteal bone resorption is present along the radial aspect of the middle phalanx, the
characteristic site for early change. There is also poor definition of the cortical outline of the tip of the
distal phalanx. The technique of magnification radiography using a fine-focus X-ray tube is helpful in
identifying these subtle appearances.

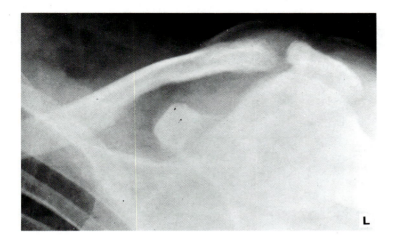

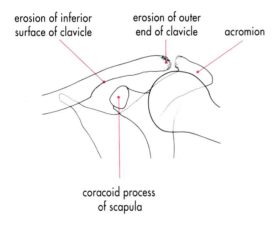

erosion of inferior
surface of clavicle

erosion of outer
end of clavicle

acromion

coracoid process
of scapula

Fig. 1.59 Primary hyperparathyroidism: erosion of the outer end of the clavicle.
This coned AP view of the lateral half of the left clavicle shows subperiosteal bone resorption of the
outer end of the clavicle with slight widening of the acromioclavicular joint. There is also erosion of the
under surface of the clavicle above the coracoid process of the scapula.

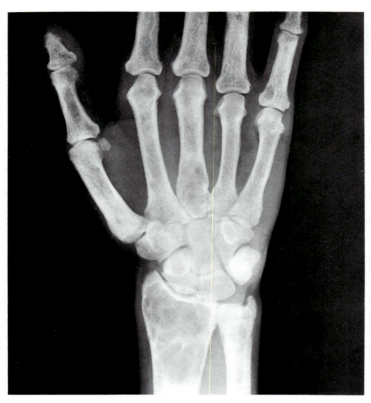

Fig. 1.60 Primary hyperparathyroidism: brown tumours. Brown tumours sometimes occur in primary hyperparathyroidism but are relatively uncommon in secondary hyperparathyroidism. This PA film of the wrist shows the typical appearance of brown tumours. Osteolucent bony defects are present in the distal radius and ulna, the base of the third metacarpal and the proximal phalanx of the little finger. The bone density is generally decreased. After parathyroidectomy brown tumours fill slowly with new bone from the periphery. Incomplete healing results in an appearance which may closely resemble that of fibrous dysplasia.

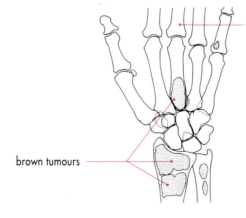

poor corticomedullary differentiation

brown tumours

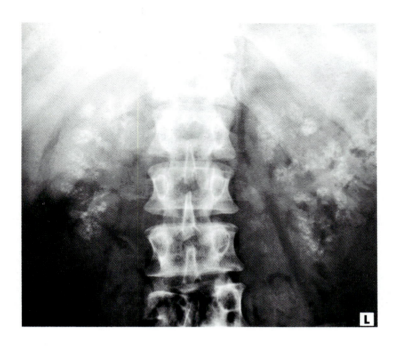

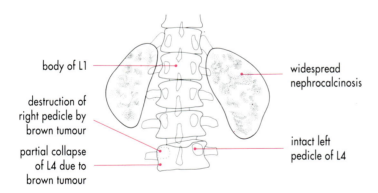

body of L1

widespread
nephrocalcinosis

destruction of
right pedicle by
brown tumour

intact left
pedicle of L4

partial collapse
of L4 due to
brown tumour

Fig. 1.61 Primary hyperparathyroidism: nephrocalcinosis and a brown tumour.
Although pathologically about 60 per cent of patients with primary hyperparathyroidism have renal
calculi or nephrocalcinosis, the radiological demonstration of such abnormalities is far less common.
This coned abdominal film shows extensive nephrocalcinosis of the fine type seen in primary
hyperparathyroidism. Generalised loss of bone density is present and a brown tumour has resulted in
the partial collapse of the body of the fourth lumbar vertebra.

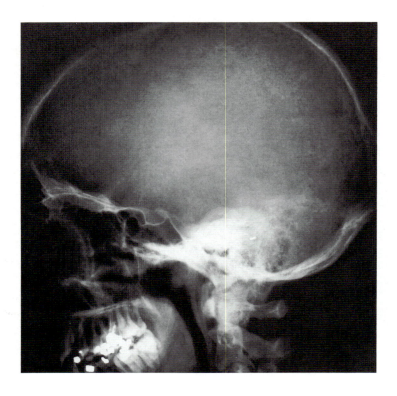

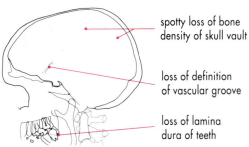

spotty loss of bone
density of skull vault

loss of definition
of vascular groove

loss of lamina
dura of teeth

Fig. 1.62 Primary hyperparathyroidism: 'pepper pot' skull. This lateral film shows
the classical changes in the skull vault of primary hyperparathyroidism. Generalised skeletal
demineralisation is reflected by diffuse porotic mottling of the calvarium giving a granular or 'pepper
pot' appearance. The vascular grooves are poorly defined and there is absence of the lamina dura of
the teeth. The latter appearance is, however, not specific because it may occur in other dimineralising
disorders such as osteoporosis and osteomalacia. In some patients with primary hyperparathyroidism
the dorsum sellae may be eroded and in those with polyglandular adenomatosis and an associated
pituitary tumour there may be enlargement of the pituitary fossa.

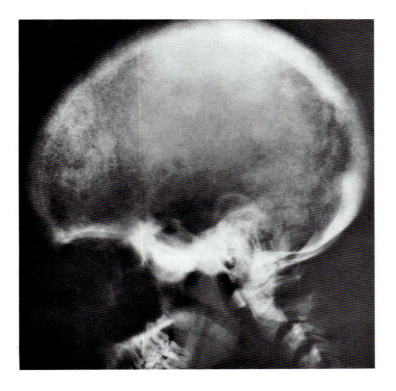

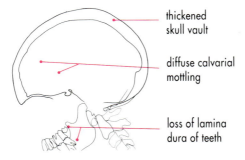

thickened
skull vault

diffuse calvarial
mottling

loss of lamina
dura of teeth

Fig. 1.63 Renal osteodystrophy: skull changes. The radiological appearances of renal osteodystrophy consist of areas of both demineralisation and sclerosis. These changes are thought to be due to a combination of osteomalacia, secondary hyperparathyroidsm and a calcitonin effect. This lateral film of the skull of a 17-year-old girl with chronic renal failure shows marked calvarial thickening with considerable mottling. Sometimes such change may resemble Paget's disease. The skull base and the cervical spine are dense and there is loss of the lamina dura of the teeth.

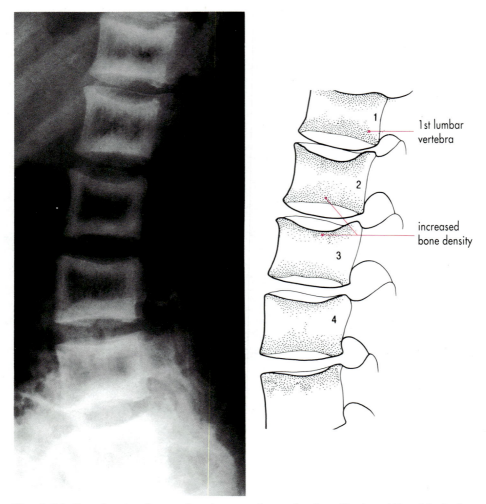

Fig. 1.64 Renal osteodystrophy: 'rugger jersey' spine. This lateral film of the lumbar spine shows central demineralisation and linear bands of subarticular density at the superior and inferior margins of the vertebral bodies – the classical appearance of a 'rugger jersey' spine.

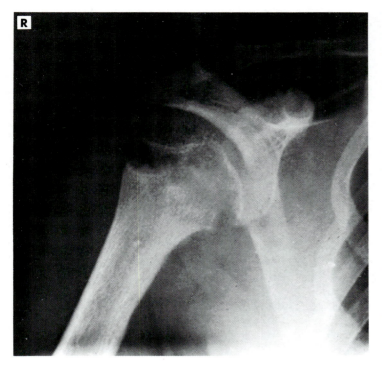

Fig. 1.65 Renal rickets: characteristic radiological appearance of the shoulder. This AP view of the right shoulder of a 16-year-old boy with chronic renal failure shows marked widening of the epiphyseal plate of the humerus with irregularity and splaying of the metaphysis characteristic features of rickets. Subperiosteal erosion of the outer end of the clavicle and of the acromion with widening of the acromioclavicular joint indicate secondary hyperparathyroidism. The bone density is generally decreased and the humeral shaft in particular demonstrates thinning of the cortex and poor definition of the corticomedullary junction. The bone age is delayed.

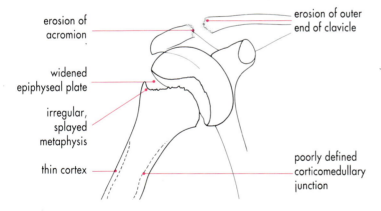

erosion of acromion

erosion of outer end of clavicle

widened epiphyseal plate

irregular, splayed metaphysis

thin cortex

poorly defined corticomedullary junction

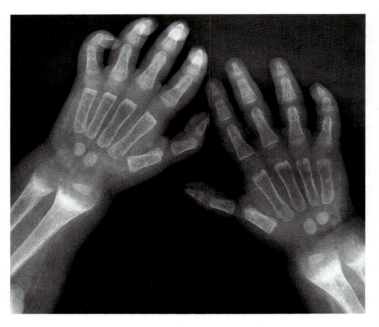

Fig. 1.66 Nutritional rickets: characteristic radiological appearance of the hands. Rickets is the term used when inadequate osteoid mineralisation affects the growing skeleton. This PA film of the hands of a two-year-old boy illustrates the characteristic appearance of nutritional rickets. Gross demineralisation of the bones is present and ossification of the secondary epiphyseal centres is delayed. Wide bands of translucency in the metaphyses and irregularity of the metaphyseal margins are characteristic. The distal radial metaphyses are cupped or splayed due to the effects of weight bearing (i.e. crawling) on the weakened bones.

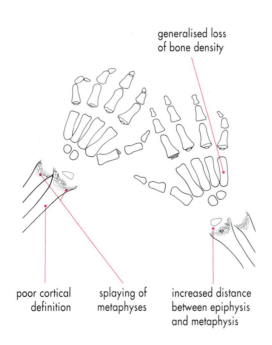

generalised loss of bone density

poor cortical definition

splaying of metaphyses

increased distance between epiphysis and metaphysis

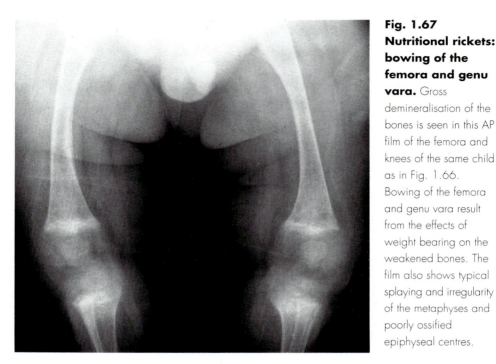

**Fig. 1.67
Nutritional rickets:
bowing of the
femora and genu
vara.** Gross
demineralisation of the
bones is seen in this AP
film of the femora and
knees of the same child
as in Fig. 1.66.
Bowing of the femora
and genu vara result
from the effects of
weight bearing on the
weakened bones. The
film also shows typical
splaying and irregularity
of the metaphyses and
poorly ossified
epiphyseal centres.

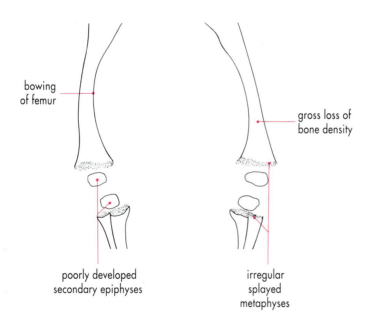

bowing
of femur

gross loss of
bone density

poorly developed
secondary epiphyses

irregular
splayed
metaphyses

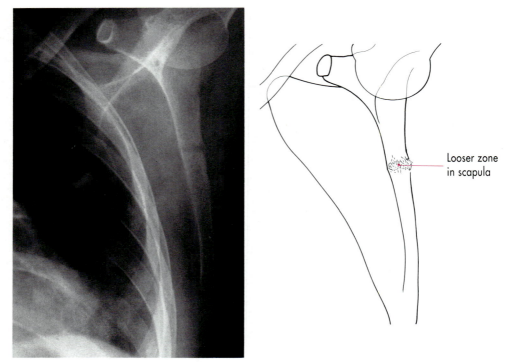

Looser zone
in scapula

Fig. 1.68 Osteomalacia: Looser zone in the scapula. Osteomalacia is the term used to describe inadequate osteoid mineralisation in the adult. Stress fractures of the weakened bones are common and the resultant seams of osteoid are known as Looser's zones. This film of the left scapula of a woman with vitamin D deficiency illustrates the typical appearance of a Looser zone. There is little or no evidence of healing. Because Looser's zones are due to stress induced by normal activity they tend to occur at constant symmetrical sites: these include the ribs, the scapulae, the obturator rings of the pelvis, the metatarsal shafts, and the femoral necks (see Fig. 1.69). Osteomalacia results in generalised demineralisation of the bones but this may be evident radiologically only when the disease is severe. When gross osteomalacia is present deformities of the weakened bones may occur: these include triradiate pelvis, kyphosis, bowing of the limbs, 'hour-glass' shaped thoracic cage and basilar invagination of the skull.

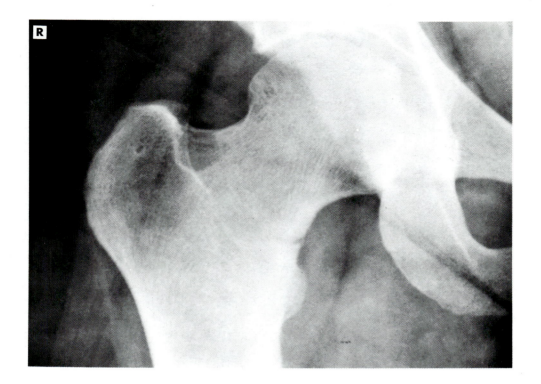

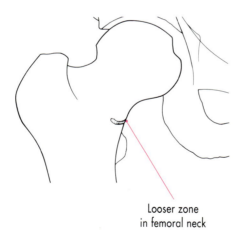

Looser zone
in femoral neck

Fig. 1.69 Osteomalacia: Looser zone in the femoral neck. This coned AP view of the upper part of the right femur shows a linear lucency in the medial aspect of the femoral neck, a typical site for a Looser zone.

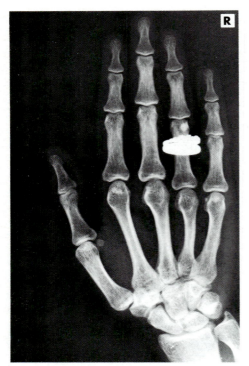

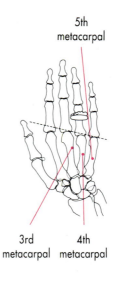

Fig. 1.70 Gonadal dysgenesis (Turner's syndrome): short fourth metacarpal. The fourth metacarpal is often short in gonadal dysgenesis, as in this patient. Normally, a line tangential to the distal ends of the third and fifth metacarpals will transect the head of the fourth. If the fourth metacarpal is short, it will touch or lie below such a line. In gonadal dysgenesis the fifth metacarpal is often also short and occasionally the third metacarpal may be similarly affected. Premature fusion of the ossification centres of the involved metacarpals may be seen in young patients.

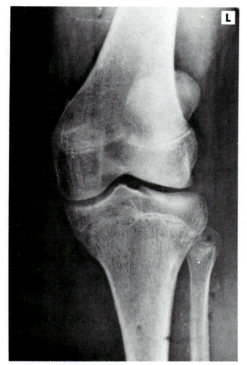

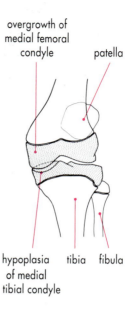

overgrowth of
medial femoral
condyle

patella

hypoplasia
of medial
tibial condyle

tibia

fibula

Fig. 1.71 Gonadal dysgenesis (Turner's syndrome): impaired development of the medial tibial condyle. This AP film of the knee shows hypoplasia of the medial tibial condyle which is often a feature of gonadal dysgenesis. The medial tibial condyle appears depressed and there is corresponding overgrowth of the medial femoral condyle.

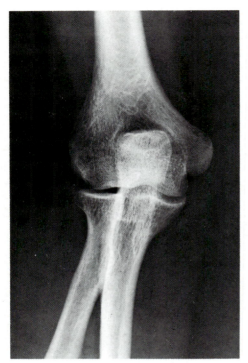
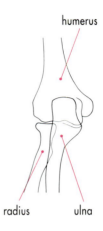

Fig. 1.72 Gonadal dysgenesis (Turner's syndrome): cubitus valgus. Bilateral cubitus valgus is frequently present in gonadal dysgenesis and this AP film of the elbow demonstrates the increase in the carrying angle, as shown by lateral deviation of the radius and ulna.

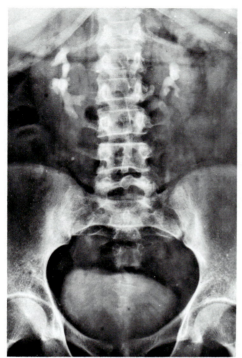

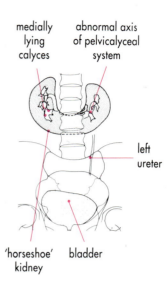

medially lying calyces

abnormal axis of pelvicalyceal system

left ureter

'horseshoe' kidney

bladder

Fig. 1.73 Gonadal dysgenesis (Turner's syndrome): fused or 'horseshoe' kidney. This full length film of an intravenous urogram shows a fused or 'horseshoe' kidney, one of the commonest associated anomalies in gonadal dysgenesis. The lower poles of the kidneys are joined in the midline and this results in abnormal orientation of the pelvicalyceal systems and medially lying calyces. Other renal anomalies, in particular those involving rotation and ectopia, are also common in gonadal dysgenesis.

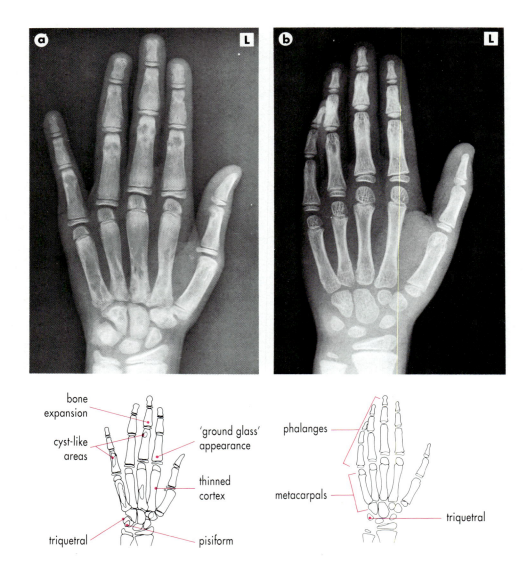

Fig. 1.74 McCune-Albright's syndrome: hand with normal for comparison. This PA film (a) of the hand of a six-year-old girl with skin pigmentation and precocious puberty shows the characteristic appearances of polyostotic fibrous dysplasia. Both bone replacement and new bone formation are evident. The affected spongiosa has an amorphous appearance resembling that of 'ground glass' and the bones show areas of expansion with thinning of the overlying cortex. Small cyst-like lesions are also present with reactive sclerosis around some of their margins. The carpal bones and secondary epiphyses are well developed and the pisiform bone, which normally starts to ossify at about nine years in the female, is seen superimposed on the triquetral. The bone age is advanced to ten years and this film should be compared with (b), that of a normal six-year-old girl, which shows the degree of bony development which usually occurs by that age.

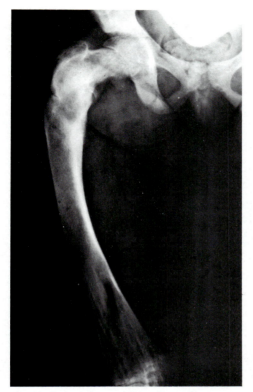

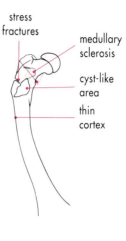

Fig. 1.75 McCune-Albright's syndrome: deformity of the femur. This AP film shows marked coxa vara and bowing of the shaft. The cyst-like lesions and areas of medullary sclerosis are typical of fibrous dysplasia. The cortex is thin, particularly at the lateral margin and stress fractures are present in the proximal femoral shaft. Such changes often progress and may result in a 'shepherd's crook' deformity of the upper femur.

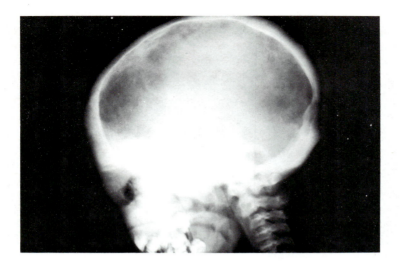

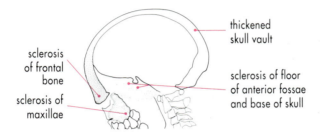

thickened
skull vault

sclerosis
of frontal
bone

sclerosis of
maxillae

sclerosis of floor
of anterior fossae
and base of skull

Fig. 1.76 McCune-Albright's syndrome: skull showing leontiasis ossea. Involvement
of the skull by fibrous dysplasia is usually manifest by extensive new bone formation and this lateral
film of the same girl as in Fig. 1.74 shows the characteristic appearance of leontiasis ossea. The
convexity of the calvarium is thickened and there is considerable sclerosis of the floor of the anterior
fossae, the base of the skull, the maxillae and the frontal bones, making the radiograph features
indistinct.

2

Imaging of the Pituitary and Hypothalamus

Robert J Witte, MD • Leighton P Mark, MD
Victor M Haughton, MD

Imaging of the pituitary and hypothalamus has evolved with the development of new imaging modalities such that pneumoencephalography and positive contrast cisternography are now only of historical interest. Although skull radiography is rarely used as a primary means of investigation of the sella it should always be evaluated when the study is obtained for other purposes (Fig. 2.1).

MAGNETIC RESONANCE IMAGING (MR)

Since its introduction, magnetic resonance imaging (MR) has taken on a major role in imaging the sella and hypothalamus. Few would argue that with its multiplanar capability and superior tissue contrast differentiation, MR imaging is the preferred initial modality, surpassing computed tomography, for patients with pituitary dysfunction or visual field defects.

MR imaging allows multiplanar images of the pituitary to be obtained with the patient's head in the neutral position. The strength of the signal depends on proton density and on two relaxation times, T1 and T2. T1 depends on the time the protons take to return to the axis of the magnetic field and T2 depends on the time the protons take to dephase. A T1-weighted image is one in which the contrast between tissues is mainly due to their T1 relaxation properties while in a T2-weighted image the contrast is due to the T2 relaxation properties. Routinely, T1-weighted images are obtained before and after intravenous contrast administration of a gadolinium chelate (i.e. gadopentatate dimeglumine). T2-weighted images are obtained when further tumour delineation or characterization is felt necessary: images are acquired in the coronal and sagittal planes.

COMPUTED TOMOGRAPHY (CT)

Computed tomography was considered for many years to be the gold standard for imaging the pituitary and hypothalamus with its high resolution and reformatting

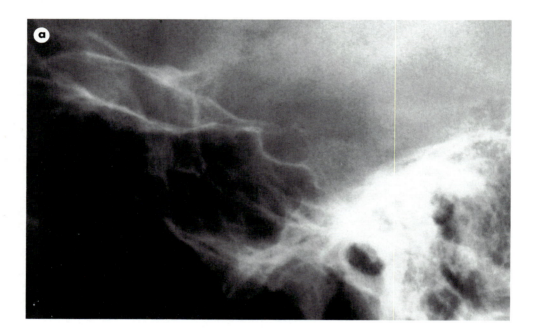

Fig. 2.1

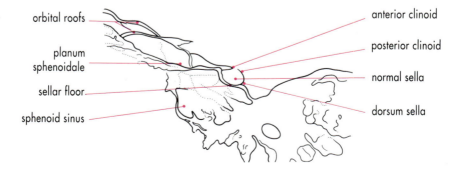

orbital roofs

planum
sphenoidale

sellar floor

sphenoid sinus

anterior clinoid

posterior clinoid

normal sella

dorsum sella

capabilities providing excellent anatomic detail of this area. Even though today MR is the preferred initial imaging modality, CT still provides a quick means to visualise thin sections of this area.

Certain patients are unable to undergo an MR examination for various reasons (e.g. a pacemaker or claustrophobia). Aneurysm clips may also be deflected in the magnetic field or may degrade MR image quality. In these patients CT still provides excellent evaluation of the sellar region. CT also provides valuable additional information to MR imaging when evaluating sellar masses with respect to bone involvement, tumour calcification and acute haemorrhage. Direct coronal images are obtained with the patient positioned in a head-holder and the neck extended comfortably to a maximal point.

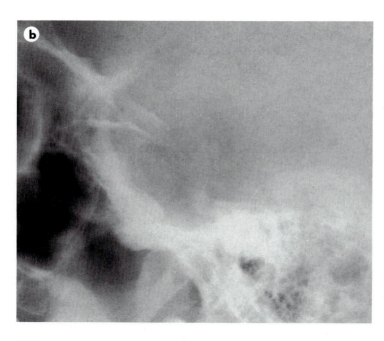

Fig. 2.1 Plain skull radiographs. Normal sella (a) and enlarged sella from pituitary macroadenoma (b).

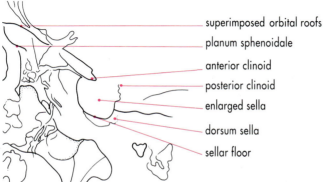

superimposed orbital roofs

planum sphenoidale

anterior clinoid

posterior clinoid

enlarged sella

dorsum sella

sellar floor

Gantry tilt is utilised to obtain an optimal coronal positioning, perpendicular to the sellar floor, while avoiding dental amalgam artefacts. A lateral localiser image is used to select contiguous coronal images, with a slice thickness of about 1.5mm. If the patient cannot be positioned for direct coronal imaging, reformatted coronal images can be obtained from axial images. Intravenous contrast medium (containing 30–40g of iodine) is administered immediately prior to the scan. Patients with a contrast allergy need to be premedicated with corticosteroids given twenty-four hours, twelve hours, and two hours prior to the study.

ANATOMY

The pituitary rests in the sella turcica, a shallow impression in the posterior sphenoid when viewed in the sagittal plane (Fig. 2.2). The anterior pituitary (adenohypophysis) accounts for about seventy-five per cent of the gland, and is the same intensity as grey matter on T1-weighted images. The contents of the posterior part of the fossa usually appear as a 'bright spot' on T1-weighted images. Proposed sources of this bright signal

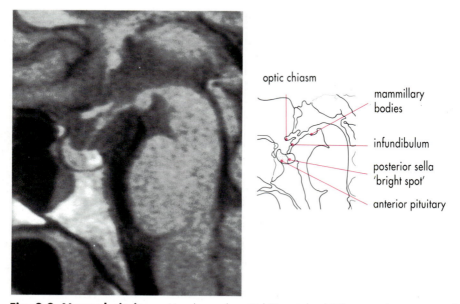

optic chiasm

mammillary bodies

infundibulum

posterior sella 'bright spot'

anterior pituitary

Fig. 2.2 Normal pituitary. Unenhanced sagittal T1-weighted MR image showing normal anatomic structures; anterior pituitary, posterior sella 'bright spot', infundibulum, optic chiasm, and mammillary bodies.

include phospholipids and/or hormones in the posterior gland (neurohypophysis) or tissue adjacent to the gland. The infundibulum can be seen extending from the tuber cinereum of the hypothalamus through the diaphragma sellae to the superior surface of the gland. The optic chiasm is anterior to, and the mammillary bodies posterior to the tuber cinereum. The midline third ventricle lies immediately above the optic chiasm and tuber cinereum.

In the coronal plane (Figs. 2.3 & 2.4), the sella is bordered laterally by the dural reflection of the cavernous sinuses. Cranial nerves III (oculomotor), IV (trochlear), V1 (ophthalmic), and V2 (maxillary) course along the lateral wall of the cavernous sinus.

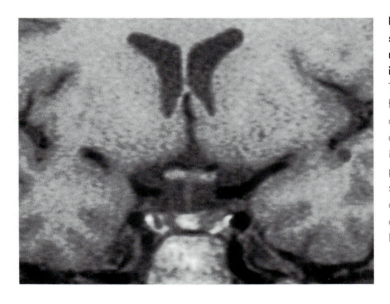

Fig. 2.3 Normal sella: magnetic resonance imaging. Coronal T1-weighted MR image following contrast administration. Normal anatomic structures include the anterior pituitary, cavernous sinus, cavernous carotid artery, infundibulum, optic chiasm and lateral ventricles.

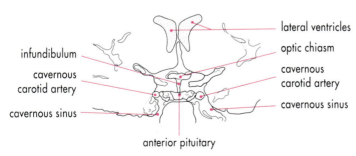

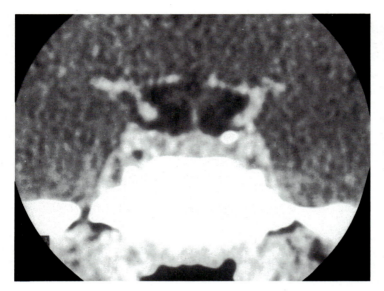

Fig. 2.4 Normal sella: computed tomography.
Normal anatomic structures include the pituitary, infundibulum, optic chiasm, cavernous sinus, internal carotid artery and middle cerebral artery.

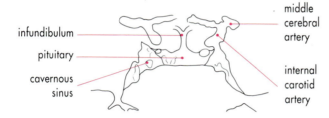

infundibulum
pituitary
cavernous sinus

middle cerebral artery
internal carotid artery

Cranial nerve VI (abducens) courses more medially along the sinus trabeculae. The pituitary stalk usually reaches the pituitary gland in the midline. However, up to forty per cent of the normal population may have an eccentric insertion. The gland usually measures 4-8mm in vertical dimension with a flat or concave superior border. The optic chiasm and third ventricle are identified superiorly, as well as the hypothalamus forming the floor of the third ventricle. Since the infundibulum and pituitary lack a blood-brain barrier, intense enhancement is seen in these structures and the cavernous sinuses following contrast administration. Mild superior glandular convexity may be seen at puberty or in lactating females (Fig. 2.5).

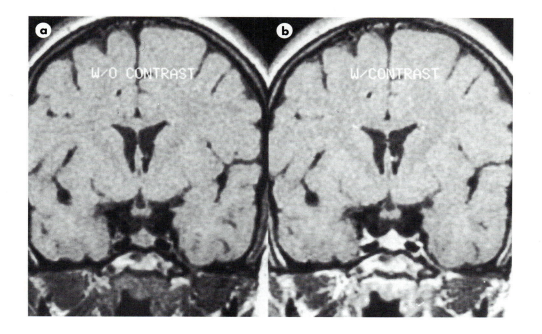

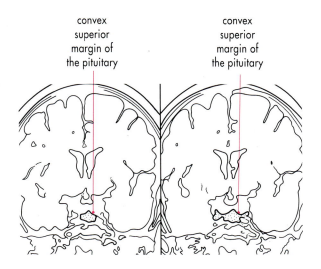

Fig. 2.5 Normal anatomic variant: magnetic resonance imaging. T1-weighted
coronal images of the sella pre-contrast administration (a) and post-contrast administration (b), show a
convex superior margin of the pituitary, a normal variant in adolescent and lactating females.

EMPTY SELLA

Defects in the diaphragma sella may allow passage of cerebrospinal fluid (CSF) from the suprasellar cistern into the sella turcica, although it may also result from infarction or irradiation of a pituitary tumour. The condition is termed 'empty sella' and is usually

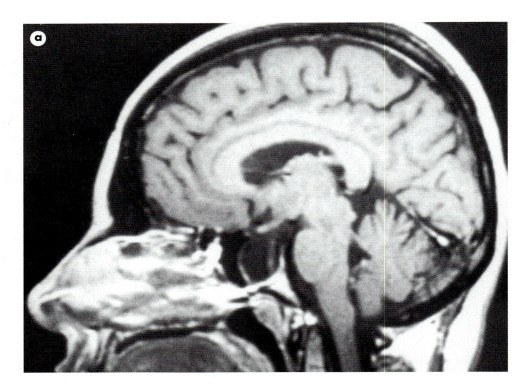

Fig. 2.6

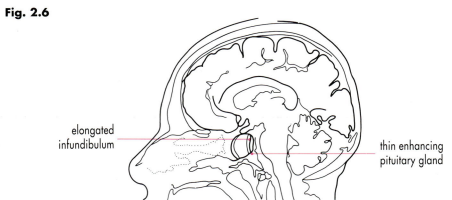

elongated infundibulum

thin enhancing pituitary gland

an incidental finding. Differentiation from an intra- or suprasellar cyst is based on the normal location of the infundibulum, extending from the tuber cinereum to a small posteriorly displaced pituitary gland (Fig. 2.6). The clinical condition of 'empty sella syndrome' has been applied to the combination of an 'empty sella' with the constellation of symptoms: headache, endocrine dysfunction, and visual disturbances.

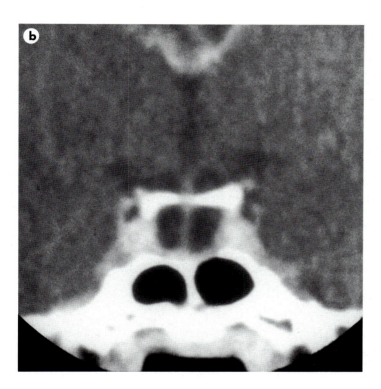

Fig. 2.6 Empty sella. Sagittal T1-weighted post-contrast MR image (a) showing a large 'empty sella', with an elongated infundibulum inserting into a thin enhancing pituitary gland. Coronal CT (b) in a different patient showing insertion of the infundibulum into a thin pituitary.

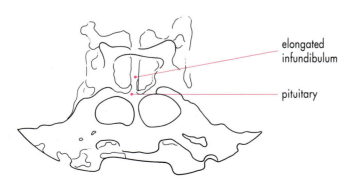

elongated
infundibulum

pituitary

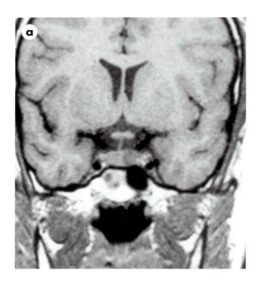

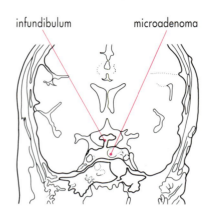

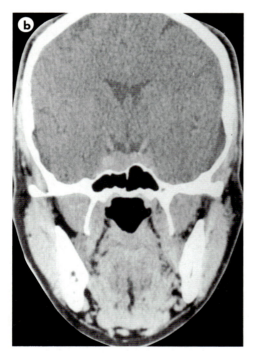

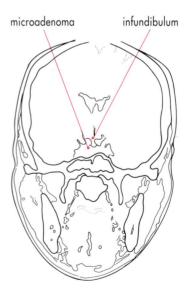

Fig. 2.7 Microadenoma. T1-weighted coronal MR image (a) showing hypointense microadenoma in the left side of the pituitary. The mass causes a convex superior margin of the gland and displacement of the infundibulum to the right. Coronal CT (b) in a different patient with a microadenoma in the right side of the pituitary displacing the infundibulum to the left.

ADENOMAS

Adenomas are classified radiographically by size. Microadenomas are considered to be less than 1cm, and macroadenomas, greater than 1cm. Microadenomas are often functional and come to clinical attention due to signs and symptoms of excess hormone secretion (i.e. prolactin, ACTH, or growth hormone). Microadenomas are usually hypointense compared with the normal pituitary on T1-weighted images. Small incidental pars intermedia cysts located between the anterior and posterior lobes may have a similar appearance or a high intensity signal. On intravenous contrast administration the microadenoma frequently enhances to a lesser degree than the surrounding gland, accentuating its hypointense appearance. Microadenomas are often asymmetrically located in the gland. Secondary signs caused by the mass effect of the microadenoma include deviation of the infundibulum away from the mass and upward convexity of the superior margin of the gland (Fig. 2.7). However, as stated above, the secondary signs are nonspecific and may be seen in the normal population. These signs are less reliable than the identification of a hypointense lesion in a symptomatic patient. A small percentage of microadenomas may show greater enhancement than the remainder of the gland following contrast administration (Fig. 2.8).

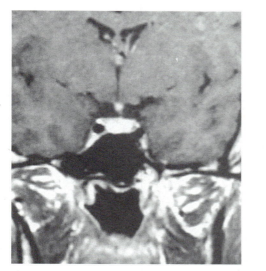
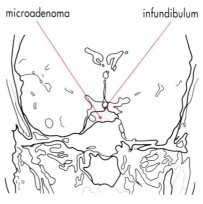

Fig. 2.8 Enhancing microadenoma: magnetic resonance imaging. Contrast enhanced T1-weighted coronal MR image showing an enhancing microadenoma in the right side of the pituitary. The infundibulum is displaced to the left.

Macroadenomas usually present clinically with signs and symptoms associated with the displacement of the optic chiasm, cavernous sinus, and hypothalamus. These tumours are often homogeneous in appearance, isointense with grey matter on T1-weighted images and enhance homogeneously after contrast administration (Fig. 2.9). Macroadenomas, however, may also be heterogeneous in appearance due to necrosis, cystic degeneration or haemorrhage. Necrotic areas show as a lower signal than the surrounding tumour on T1-weighted images. Areas that progress to cystic degeneration show as a signal which is similar to CSF (i.e. low on T1-weighted images and high on T2-weighted images). Acute haemorrhage in these tumours is best seen as high density areas on non-contrasted CT studies whilst subacute haemorrhage is easier to identify using MR studies, appearing as high signal on T1-weighted images.

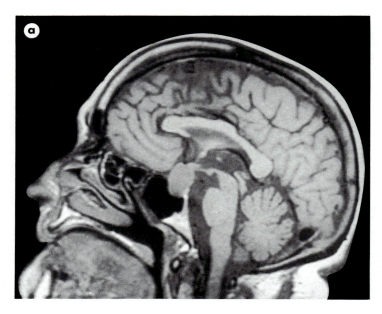

Fig. 2.9
Macroadenoma.
Sagittal T1-weighted MR image (a) showing a large sellar/suprasellar macroadenoma. Coronal image (b) following contrast administration shows diffuse homogeneous enhancement with upward displacement of the optic chiasm more clearly identified. Coronal CT (c) of a macroadenoma in a different patient also demonstrating diffuse homogeneous enhancement.

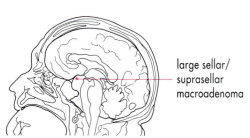

large sellar/
suprasellar
macroadenoma

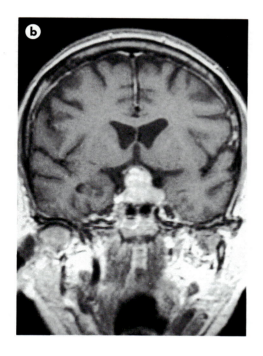

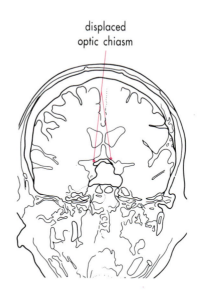

displaced
optic chiasm

Fig. 2.9

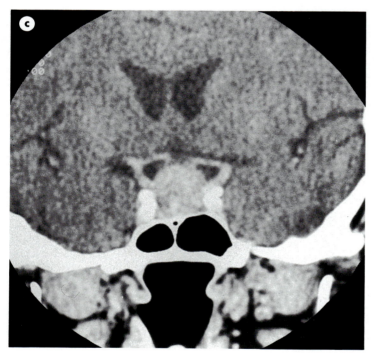

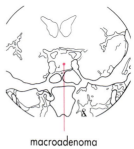

macroadenoma

Macroadenoma appearance on T2-weighted images varies (Fig. 2.10). A region of high signal intensity would suggest necrosis. Calcification, although rare, may also be seen and is usually curvilinear.

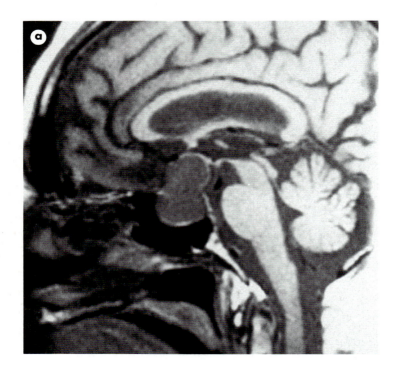

Fig. 2.10

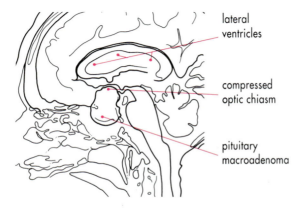

lateral
ventricles

compressed
optic chiasm

pituitary
macroadenoma

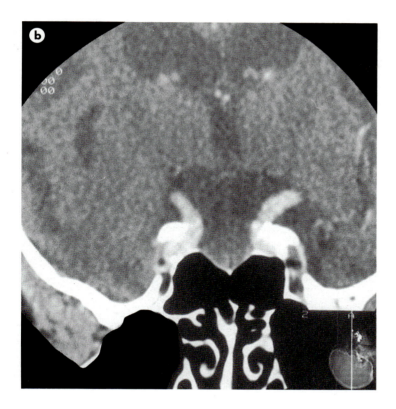

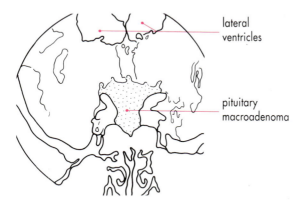

Fig. 2.10 Cystic macroadenoma. Sagittal T1-weighted MR image (a) showing a large pituitary macroadenoma with suprasellar extension, compressing the optic chiasm. The low signal intensity of the mass is similar to the CSF signal in the lateral ventricles suggesting the predominantly cystic nature of the mass. A coronal CT (b) in the same patient showing the mass to be of low density, like the CSF in the lateral ventricles.

Extrasellar extension of macroadenoma has important clinical and surgical implications. Suprasellar extension may produce a 'waist' due to compression by the diaphragma sellae (Fig. 2.11). CT best evaluates erosion of the sellar floor and inferior extension into the sphenoid sinus and sphenoid extension is suggested by the appearance of a convex inferior margin of the mass on CT and MR images. However, cavernous sinus extension, particularly when early, is difficult to detect. Unilateral encasement of the carotid artery and distortion of the lateral margins of the cavernous sinus are the most reliable signs (see Fig. 2.11 (b) & (c)).

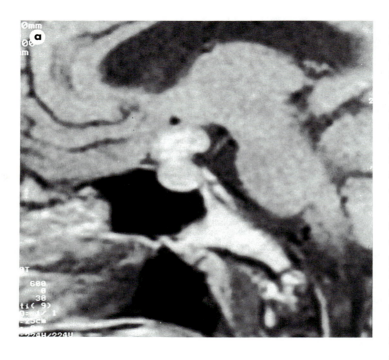

Fig. 2.11 Extrasellar extension of macroadenomas. Sagittal T1-weighted MR image (a) showing suprasellar extension with a 'waist' caused by the diaphragma sellae. Coronal T1-weighted MR image (b) demonstrating suprasellar and left cavernous sinus extension, encasing the left cavernous carotid artery. Coronal CT image (c) showing suprasellar, cavernous sinus, and sphenoid sinus extension.

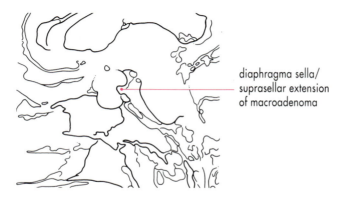

diaphragma sella/ suprasellar extension of macroadenoma

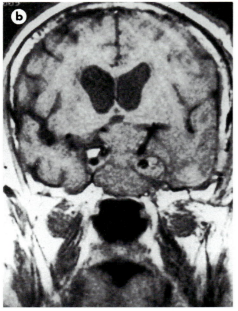

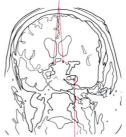

suprasellar extension
of macroadenoma

left cavernous
sinus extension of
macroadenoma

Fig. 2.11

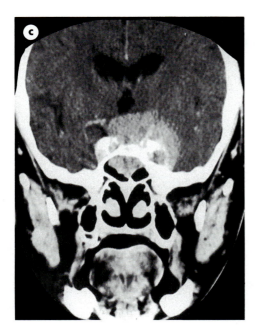

suprasellar
extension

cavernous
sinus extension of
macroadenoma

sphenoid sinus
extension of
macroadenoma

Post-partum pituitary haemorrhagic infarction may lead to hypopituitarism (Sheehan's syndrome). This appears radiographically as a dense gland on CT examination (Fig. 2.12).

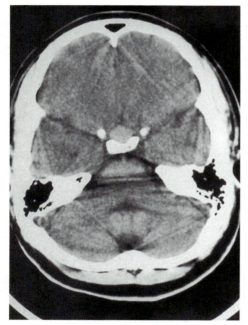

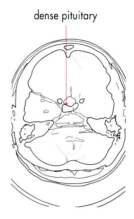

Fig. 2.12 Sheehan's syndrome: computed tomography. Axial CT image showing a dense pituitary due to haemorrhagic infarction following uterine haemorrhage post-partum.

Adenomas in other patients may also undergo haemorrhagic infarction. The enlarged haemorrhagic gland may be dysfunctional and compress adjacent structures, producing pituitary apoplexy (Fig. 2.13).

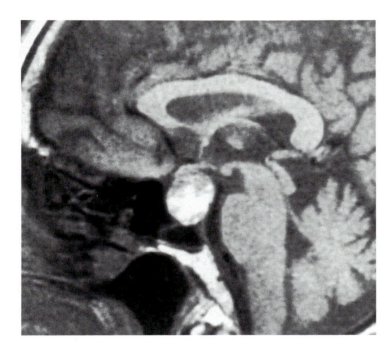

Fig. 2.13 Pituitary apoplexy: magnetic resonance imaging. T1-weighted sagittal MR image showing haemorrhage in a macroadenoma.

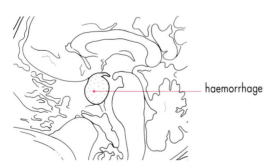

haemorrhage

MENINGIOMAS

Meningiomas are the second most common tumour in the sellar region. These tumours may arise from dural surfaces such as the diaphragma sellae, tuberculum sellae, or cavernous sinuses. These tumours may project into the suprasellar space and rarely arise within the sella. These tumours are usually isointense with grey matter on T1- and T2-

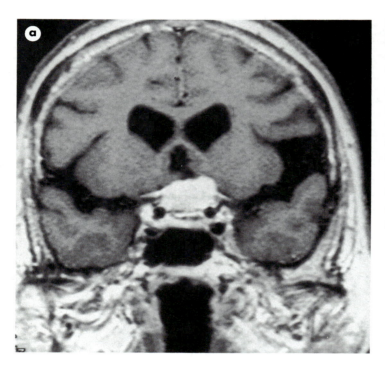

Fig. 2.14
Meningioma.
Contrast-enhanced, T1-weighted coronal MR image (a) demonstrating an enhancing suprasellar meningioma with adjacent 'dural tail'. Coronal CT image (b) in a different patient also demonstrating an enhancing suprasellar meningioma.

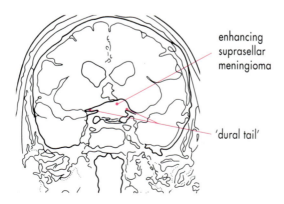

enhancing
suprasellar
meningioma

'dural tail'

weighted images and enhance intensely following contrast administration. Differentiation from an adenoma with suprasellar extension may be difficult. A dural 'tail' sign may be produced by adjacent dural enhancement (Fig. 2.14). Coronal images are very helpful in distinguishing the purely suprasellar location of the meningioma from the intrasellar and suprasellar location of the adenoma.

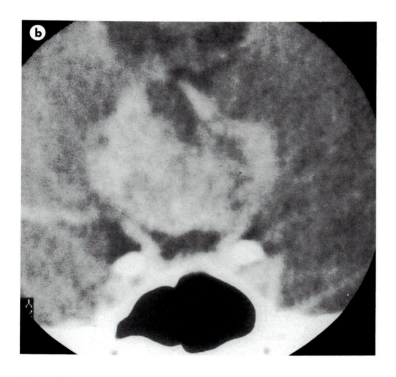

Fig. 2.14

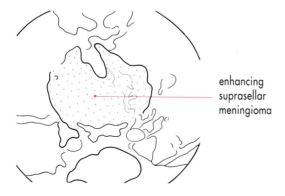

enhancing
suprasellar
meningioma

CRANIOPHARYNGIOMAS

Craniopharyngiomas are benign neoplasms which may arise from epithelial remnants of Rathké's pouch. They are the most frequent neoplasm in the sellar region in children and young adults. A second peak also occurs in adults at around the fifth decade.

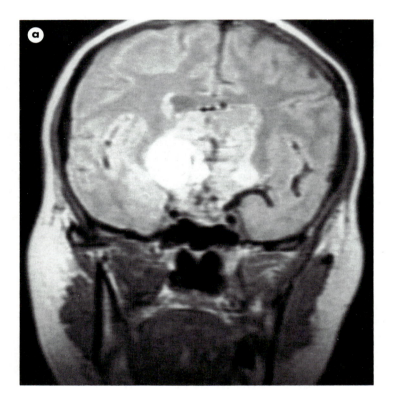

Fig. 2.15

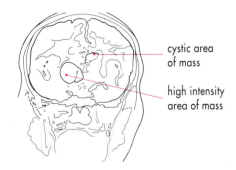

cystic area
of mass

high intensity
area of mass

These tumours usually arise in the suprasellar region, however, they may be both suprasellar and intrasellar, or entirely intrasellar. Craniopharyngiomas are radiographically heterogeneous in appearance, often containing cysts and globular calcification (Fig. 2.15). The cystic portions of the mass may appear hypointense on T1-weighted MR images, and hyperintense on T2-weighted images. Craniopharyngiomas may also

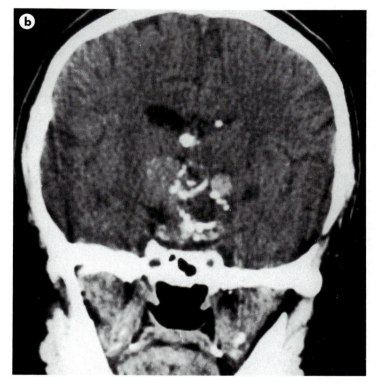

**Fig. 2.15
Craniopharyngioma.**
Balanced-weighted coronal MR image (a) showing a cystic area and high intensity signal area in a large sellar/suprasellar mass, typical of craniopharyngiomas. Characteristic globular calcification is easier to identify on a coronal CT image (b) of the same patient.

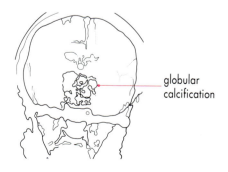

globular
calcification

exhibit both iso- and hyperintense components. The solid portions of the mass, and the periphery of the cystic components often enhance following contrast administration. MR imaging best shows the mass to be anatomically separate from the pituitary, helping to differentiate the mass from an adenoma. The calcification is much more

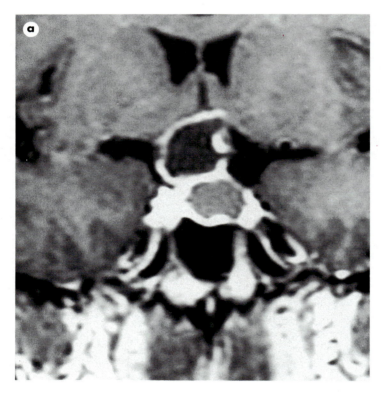

Fig. 2.16 Atypical craniopharyngioma. Coronal T1-weighted MR image (a) following contrast administration showing enhancement of a solid sellar mass with a ring enhancing suprasellar cystic component. A CT image (b) of the same patient shows a ring of calcification around the cystic portion of the mass.

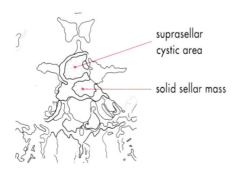

suprasellar cystic area

solid sellar mass

apparent on CT examination which is often useful in differentiation from other masses. Less commonly, these tumours may appear entirely solid or demonstrate ring calcification surrounding a cystic component (Fig. 2.16).

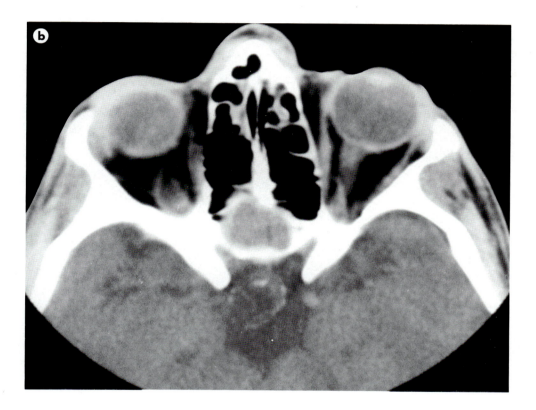

Fig. 2.16

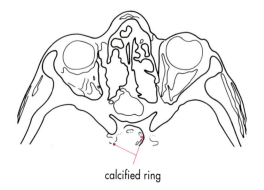

calcified ring

ANEURYSMS

Aneurysms of the intracavernous or supraclinoid carotid artery appear as a dense sellar or juxtasellar masses on CT imaging, with enhancement following contrast administration. However, differentiation from a true neoplasm is often difficult. These lesions are also easily identified on conventional MR examination but unlike stationary tissue, rapidly flowing blood produces little signal. Therefore, MR angiography is another technique that can be used to identify aneurysms (Fig. 2.17).

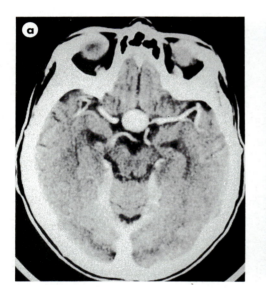
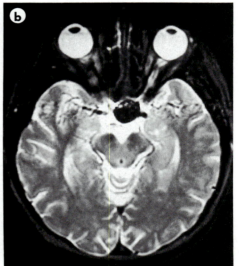

Fig. 2.17

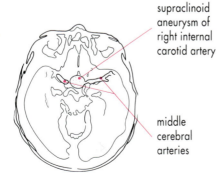
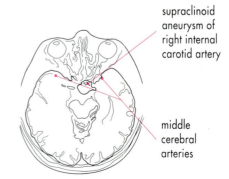

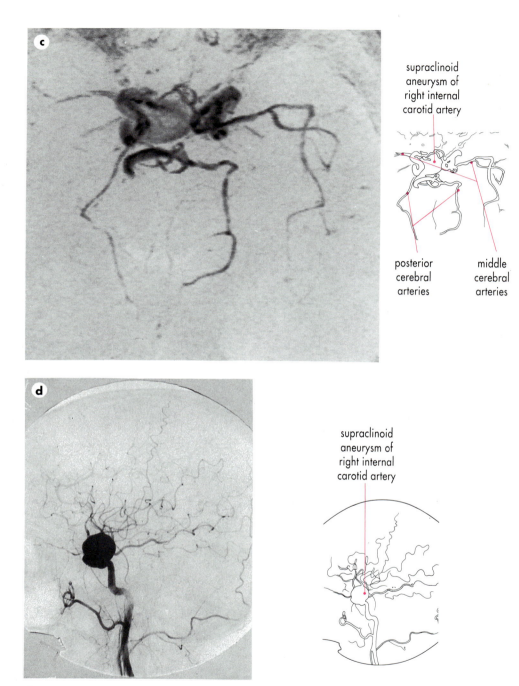

Fig. 2.17 Supraclinoid aneurysm. Multiple studies of the same patient showing a supraclinoid aneurysm of the right internal carotid artery. The middle cerebral arteries are also demonstrated: (a) enhanced CT image; (b) T2-weighted MR image; (c) MR angiogram of similar orientation to (a) and (b), posterior cerebral arteries are also identified; (d) cerebral angiogram.

GLIOMAS

Gliomas occurring in the sellar region primarily involve the hypothalamus and optic chiasm. Hypothalamic gliomas are tumours of childhood and adolescence, and may extend into the suprasellar cistern. Chiasmic gliomas have a strong association with neurofibromatosis type I when occurring in children. They appear as sharply margin-ated homogeneous suprasellar masses, clearly separate from the pituitary gland. They are also usually hypointense or isointense with grey matter and may or may not enhance (Fig. 2.18).

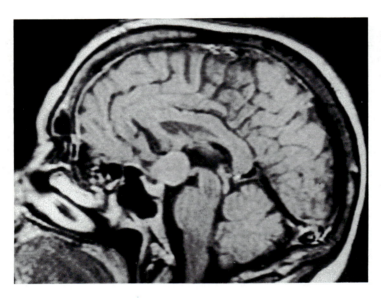

Fig. 2.18 Chiasmic glioma: magnetic resonance imaging. T1-weighted sagittal MR image showing chiasmic glioma displacing mammillary bodies posteriorly. Note the normal pituitary gland.

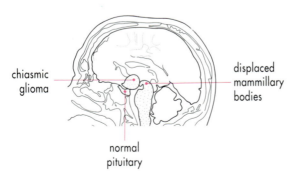

chiasmic glioma

displaced mammillary bodies

normal pituitary

CHORDOMAS

Chordomas are neoplasms that develop from intraosseous vestigial remnants of the notochord. The sacrum is the most common site accounting or fifty per cent of occurrences, followed by the clivus at thirty-five per cent. Clival chordomas may project into the sella or suprasellar regions. MR and CT techniques are both important in the differential diagnosis of these tumours. MR imaging best shows tumour infiltration and tumour origin in the clivus. Characteristic tumoural calcification is better identified with CT imaging. These tumours are often slightly hypointense on T1-weighted MR images and intensely enhanced following contrast administration (Fig. 2.19). Chondrosarcomas of the clivus may have an identical appearance on CT and MR studies.

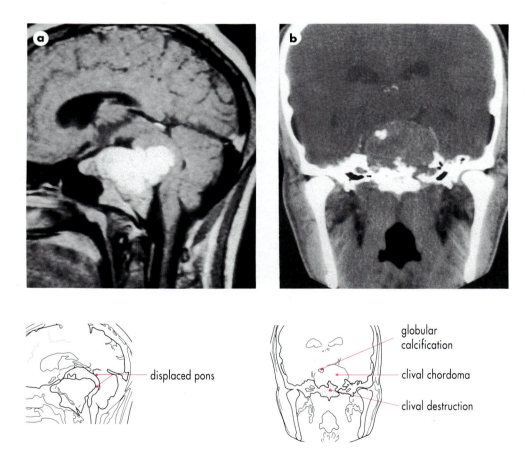

Fig. 2.19 Clival chordoma. Contrast enhanced T1-weighted sagittal MR image (a) showing an intensely enhancing large clival chordoma. The tumour compresses and displaces the pons posteriorly. Coronal CT image (b) in the same patient demonstrating globular calcification within the mass and clival destruction.

CYSTS

Arachnoid cysts may arise in the suprasellar cistern, or adjacent parasellar regions. Remnants of Rathké's pouch may produce midline epithelial cysts termed Rathké's cleft cysts. These cysts may produce hydrocephalus or compress the optic chiasm, pituitary or infundibulum. These lesions may be difficult to identify because their signal intensities in MR imaging or density in CT is identical to CSF (Fig. 2.20). Rathké's cleft cysts, however, may be hyperintense to CSF on T1-weighted MR images. The diagnosis of arachnoid cysts is made radiologically by noting displacement of the pituitary stalk, chiasm or base of the brain.

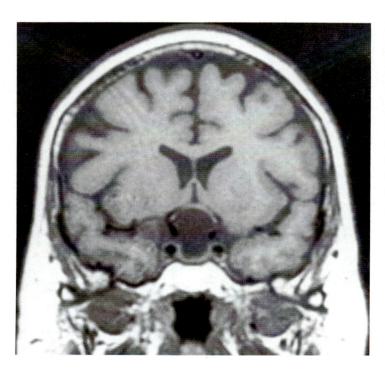

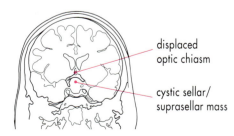

Fig. 2.20 Sellar cyst: magnetic resonance imaging. T1-weighted coronal MR image showing a cystic sellar/suprasellar mass and displacement of the optic chiasm. Absence of an identifiable infundibulum differentiates this mass from an 'empty sella'.

displaced optic chiasm

cystic sellar/ suprasellar mass

INFLAMMATORY DISEASE

Tuberculosis and sarcoidosis may involve the CNS, producing suprasellar masses or thickening of the infundibulum or optic chiasm. These granulomatous lesions are usually isointense with grey matter on T1-weighted MR images. Enhancement of the parenchymal lesions, as well as leptomeningeal enhancement are seen following contrast administration (Fig. 2.21). Other causes of infundibular thickening include lymphoma, metastatic carcinoma, and Langerhans' cell histiocytosis (histiocytosis X) (Fig. 2.22).

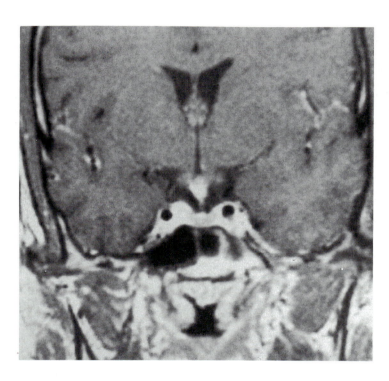

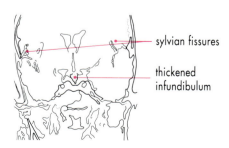

Fig. 2.21 Sarcoidosis: magnetic resonance imaging. Coronal T1-weighted image following contrast administration shows a thickened, enhancing infundibulum typical of CNS granulomatous disease. Enhancement in both sylvian fissures identifies leptomeningeal involvement.

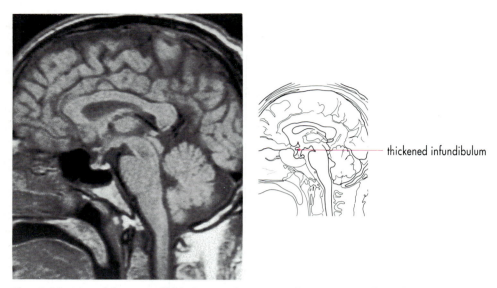

thickened infundibulum

Fig. 2.22 Langerhans' cell histiocytosis: magnetic resonance imaging. Sagittal T1-weighted MR image showing a thickened infundibulum from known histiocytosis.

EXOPHTHALMOS

There are many causes of exophthalmos, however, the majority of cases are due to Graves' disease in adults. MR provides optimal imaging of the orbits, with coronal and axial planes obtained with the patient's head in the neutral position. CT can also be used for orbital imaging by utilizing thin slices (3mm) in the axial and direct coronal planes.

The most common presentation is bilateral and symmetric ocular muscle enlargement with preference for the inferior and medial rectus. Bilateral asymmetric and occasionally unilateral involvement can also occur (Fig. 2.23). Idiopathic inflammation or 'inflammatory pseudotumour' is another frequent cause of exophthalmos which often causes ocular muscle enlargement. Involvement is usually unilateral and tends to involve the muscles' tendinous insertion into the globe or may even present as an

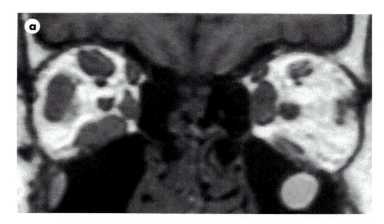

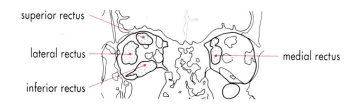

superior rectus

lateral rectus

inferior rectus

medial rectus

Fig. 2.23
Endocrine
ophthalmopathy.
Coronal T1-weighted
MR image (a) showing
extraocular muscle
enlargement of the
superior rectus, lateral
rectus and inferior
rectus of the right orbit.
Enlargement of the
medial rectus in the left
orbit is also present.
Coronal CT (b) in a
different patient with
enlargement of the
medial rectus and
superior rectus of both
orbits.

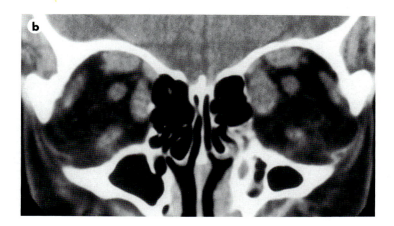

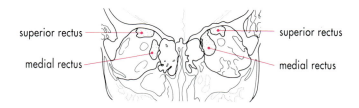

superior rectus

superior rectus

medial rectus

medial rectus

orbital mass. Other causes for exophthalmos are usually unilateral and include benign and malignant tumours (Fig. 2.24), vascular malformations, carotid-cavernous fistula, or cavernous sinus thrombosis.

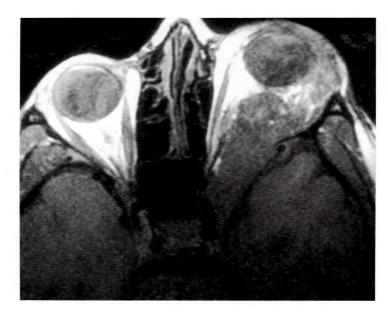

Fig. 2.24 Neurofibroma: magnetic resonance imaging. Large neurofibroma of the left orbit causing exophthalmos of the left globe.

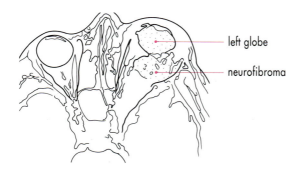

left globe

neurofibroma

3

Nuclear Medicine Imaging In Endocrinology

Keith E Britton, MD, MSc, FRCP • Jamshed B Bomanji, MD, MSc, PhD

Nuclear medicine is to physiology what radiology is to anatomy. For imaging in endocrinology an agent is chosen whose uptake or metabolism relates to the function of the particular endocrine system. The agent is radiolabelled with a γ-emitting radionuclide so that, after its intravenous or oral administration, it can be detected externally and noninvasively by imaging with a γ-camera. Nuclear medicine techniques may also characterise a tissue by its receptor or antigen expression in ways complementary to radiological and biochemical techniques. It allows in vivo assessment of clinical physiology and pathophysiology and is very sensitive to metabolic disorders. Furthermore, stimulation and suppression techniques can be used to enhance its specificity. The absorbed radiation dose equivalent to the patients from diagnostic tests is of the same order as from X-ray studies; usually up to 7.5mSv (0.75rem). One sievert (Sv) equals one hundred radiation dose equivalents (rem). Natural background radiation from cosmic rays, body potassium, radon, etc. is, in London, about 2mSv (0.2rem) and in Cornwall, 8mSv (0.8rem) annually. Thus, these tests give activities that are considered by the International Committee of Radiation Protection to be of negligible risk to members of the public (up to 5mSv) and to workers using ionising radiation (up to 15mSv).

For therapy, the destructive properties of β-particle (electron) emitting radionuclides are used, so that radiation therapy can be targeted by the chosen carrier agent to the site of the disorder or cancer. This facilitates delivery of therapeutic levels of radiation even more selectively than is possible by external beam therapy.

a

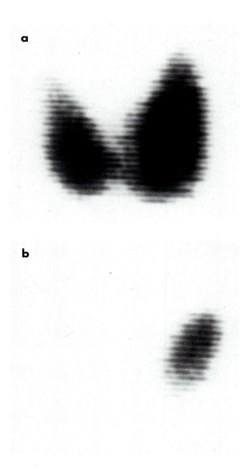

b

Fig. 3.1 Thyroid images in thyrotoxicosis. These are obtained by γ-camera imaging of the anterior neck 20 minutes after intravenous injection of 80MBq ⁹⁹ᵐTc pertechnetate. ⁹⁹ᵐTc pertechnetate is trapped but not organified, while radioiodine is trapped and organified by the thyroid gland. (a) Typical image in Graves' disease with homogeneously increased uptake in an enlarged gland; in this case the left lobe is bigger than the right lobe. (b) Typical appearance in an autonomous toxic nodule (Plummer's syndrome) with suppression of uptake in the remaining normal thyroid. (c) Typical appearance of a toxic multinodular goitre with areas of autonomous toxic nodules separated by areas of nodules with no function and areas of normal tissue whose function has been suppressed.

c

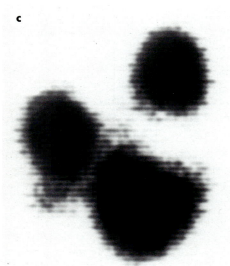

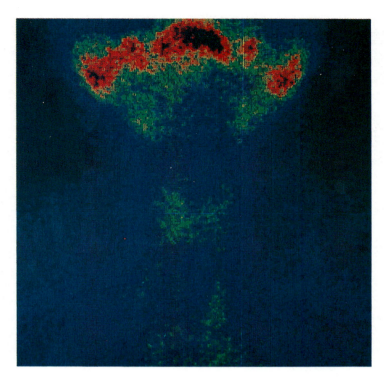

Fig. 3.2 Hyperthyroidism due to subacute thyroiditis. ^{99m}Tc pertechnetate images taken 20 minutes after injection. Using the colour scale 0–100% (blue - green - yellow - red - purple) the thyroid can be seen in green, at the same level as the vascular activity in the aorta and heart inferiorly. Uptake is much reduced below that in the salivary glands and mouth seen superiorly. Normally, thyroid uptake is greater than salivary gland uptake. In this case, with clinical hyperthyroidism, there is severe reduction of uptake due to the inflammation of the thyroid. Autoimmune thyroiditis is a great mimic of the range of thyroid scan abnormalities, from the Hashimoto goitre with inhomogeneous uptake to appearances of 'warm' or 'cold' defects, solitary or multiple, or asymmetric uptake.

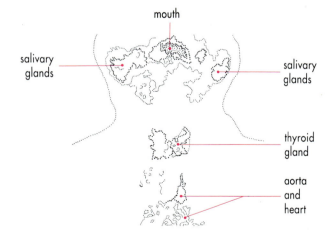

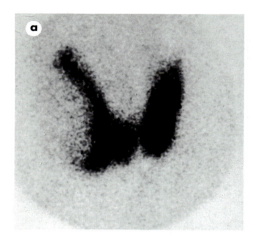

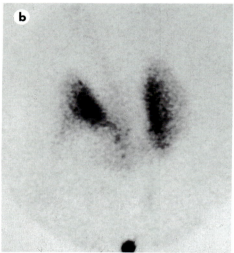

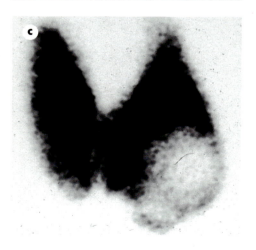

Fig. 3.3 Thyroid images in patients with palpable solitary nodules in their thyroid glands. You will note that the appearances of the scans are similar, each showing an area of deficient or reduced uptake while the rest of the gland shows a homogeneous normal uptake. It is not possible to distinguish between the causes of a solitary nodule: (a) a haemorrhage, (b) a cyst, (c) a follicular thyroid cancer. Ultrasound should be combined with thyroid imaging to demonstrate the simple cyst for aspiration cytology, and to enable fine-needle biopsy for the echogenic (solid) nodule, which is nonfunctional in a thyroid scan. If the mass in the gland is solitary and solid, about 12 per cent of these cases prove to be malignant.

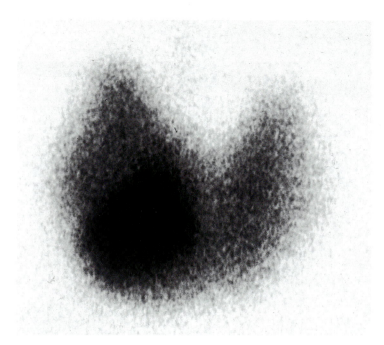

Fig. 3.4 A 'warm' nodule imaged using ^{99m}Tc pertechnetate.
Uptake in the inferior pole of the enlarged right lobe of the thyroid is greater than that in the surrounding gland and corresponds to the site of a palpable nodule. The study should be repeated using ^{123}I; see scheme in Fig. 3.5.

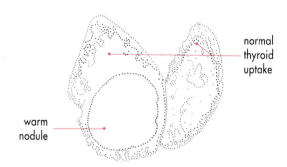

normal
thyroid
uptake

warm
nodule

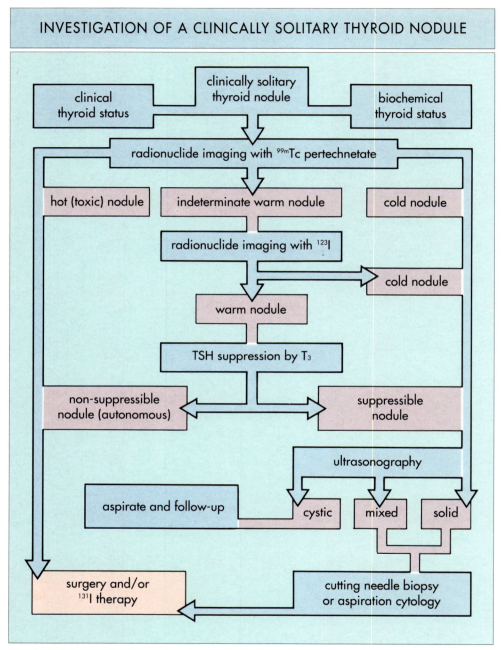

INVESTIGATION OF A CLINICALLY SOLITARY THYROID NODULE

clinical thyroid status

clinically solitary thyroid nodule

biochemical thyroid status

radionuclide imaging with ^{99m}Tc pertechnetate

hot (toxic) nodule

indeterminate warm nodule

cold nodule

radionuclide imaging with ^{123}I

cold nodule

warm nodule

TSH suppression by T$_3$

non-suppressible nodule (autonomous)

suppressible nodule

ultrasonography

aspirate and follow-up

cystic

mixed

solid

surgery and/or ^{131}I therapy

cutting needle biopsy or aspiration cytology

Fig. 3.5 Scheme for investigating a clinically solitary thyroid nodule. It should be noted that the cytopathologist can identify anaplastic, papillary and medullary carcinoma and lymphoma on aspiration biopsy. It is not possible on cytological smears to differentiate follicular adenomas from follicular carcinomas since the latter require identification of vascular invasion for diagnosis.

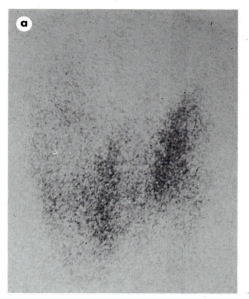

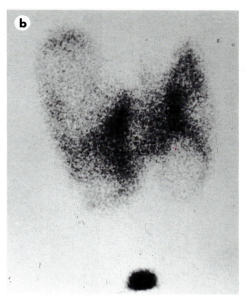

Fig. 3.6 Thyroid imaging in a patient with a multinodular goitre. (a) Using 80MBq
^{99m}Tc pertechnetate and (b) using 20MBq ^{123}I sodium iodide. The typical mix of areas of reduced
uptake and normal uptake is seen corresponding to the palpable nodules. The incidence of cancer in
such a thyroid is low. However, a dominant nonfunctional nodule should be evaluated as a solitary
'cold' nodule.

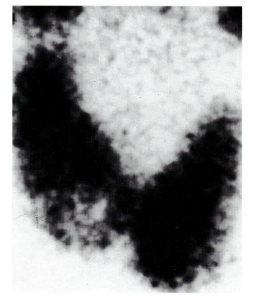

**Fig. 3.7 Thyroid image in thyrotoxicosis
in a patient with a palpable nodule.**
This image shows the uniform high uptake seen in
Graves' disease with an area of reduced uptake
('cold' area) in the inferior pole of the right thyroid
lobe. The incidence of malignancy in a solitary
'cold' nodule in a thyrotoxic gland is greater than
that in a euthyroid gland.

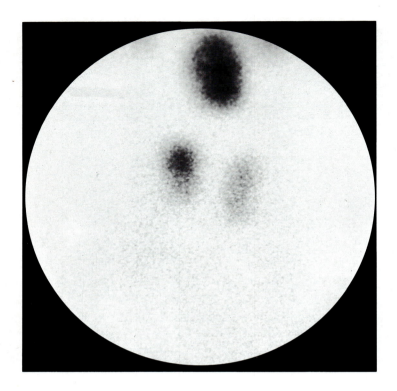

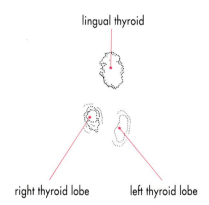

lingual thyroid

right thyroid lobe   left thyroid lobe

Fig. 3.8 Thyroid images in sublingual thyroid. This seventy-seven-year-old woman presented with a mass at the back of her tongue. Thyroid ^{99m}Tc pertechnetate imaging shows this to be a source of high uptake. Relatively reduced uptake is seen in the normal thyroid position. Thyroid scanning is an important method for evaluating lumps at the back of the tongue and in the centre of the neck. If there is a doubt about pertechnetate uptake which vascular lesions can mimic, then ^{123}I should be used. A typical thyroglossal cyst is nonfunctional on a thyroid scan.

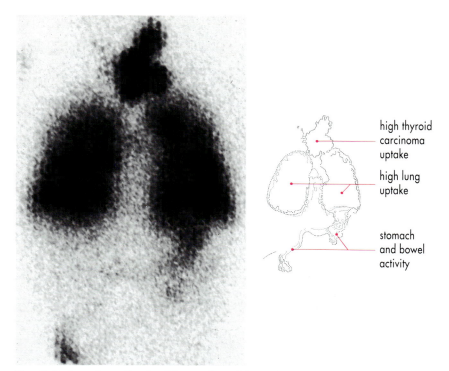

high thyroid
carcinoma
uptake

high lung
uptake

stomach
and bowel
activity

**Fig. 3.9 Functionally significant thyroid carcinoma imaged three days after
[131]I therapy (150 mCi, 5.55 GBq).** In this case, imaging shows irregular increased uptake in
the superior mediastinum, in the paratracheal and supraclavicular nodes, and diffuse high lung uptake.
Such uptake may occur rarely when there is a normal chest X-ray, but is usually associated with miliary
lung metastases and shows a good response to ^{131}I therapy. High lung uptake may be followed by
radiation fibrosis if the dose administered is too great. Indications for ^{131}I therapy are biopsy proven
papillary or follicular carcinoma and known or suspected incomplete surgical excision. Differentiated
tumours concentrate ^{131}I better than undifferentiated and Hürthle cell cancers. Thyroid carcinoma
tissue, which at first appears to take up ^{131}I poorly, may show significant uptake of tracer when all the
higher avidity normal gland has been ablated.

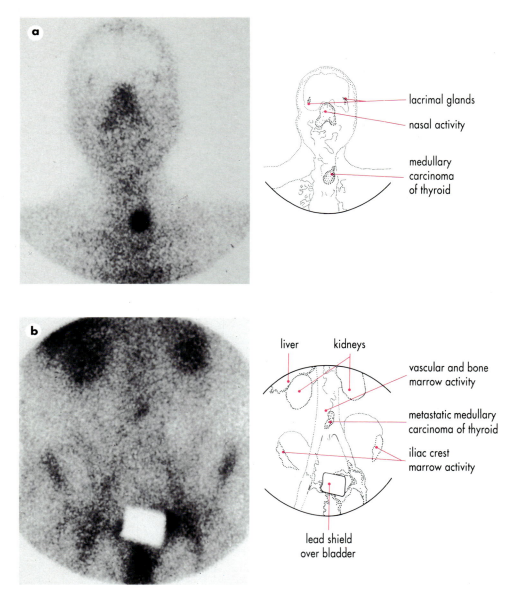

Fig. 3.10 Medullary carcinoma of the thyroid (MCT) imaged with ⁹⁹ᵐTc dimercaptosuccinic acid (DMSA-V). These images were taken four hours after intravenous injection of ⁹⁹ᵐTc DMSA-V. In (a) the head and neck have focally increased uptake in the region of the thyroid to the left of the midline. Note normal thyroid tissue is not shown. Image of the anterior abdomen (b); in the centre of the abdomen a small area of increased uptake is seen which was subsequently shown to be a metastasis of the MCT. ⁹⁹ᵐTc DMSA-V is taken up by several other tumours and by some types of amyloid. Its most consistent uptake is in MCT and it is used to demonstrate primary and recurrent disease. MCT does not take up radioiodine or ⁹⁹ᵐTc pertechnetate and appears as a 'cold' area on a conventional thyroid scan.

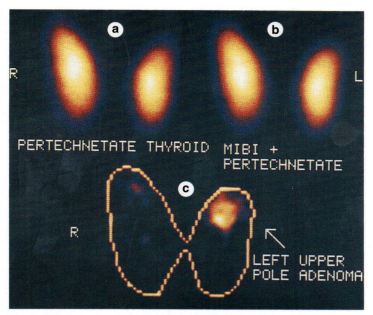

Fig. 3.11 Imaging of a parathyroid adenoma. Image (a) shows a pertechnetate thyroid scan obtained conventionally 10–20 minutes after the intravenous injection of ^{99m}Tc pertechnetate through an indwelling needle. Without the patient moving, ^{99m}Tc methoxyisobutylisonitrile (MIBI) is injected and a further series of images taken. In (b) ^{99m}Tc MIBI is taken up both by the parathyroid adenoma and by normal thyroid so that a combined composite image is seen. Using a change detection algorithm, the change between the two images is determined and the statistical degree of that difference is plotted as a probability. In (c) the high red and orange in the upper pole of the left lobe of the thyroid indicates a change between the two images with a significance of over one in a thousand. This is the site of the upper pole parathyroid adenoma. The outline of the thyroid is also shown. A small area of increased probability of change is also seen in the upper pole of the right lobe of the thyroid. Subsequently a left upper pole thyroid adenoma was removed and a right upper pole hyperplastic gland (100mg) was also removed. Prior to imaging, it is important biochemically to confirm that hypercalcaemia is due to hyperparathyroidism. Imaging of the parathyroid is intended to localise the site of adenomas or hyperplastic glands. Visualisation of a gland depends upon its size. A normal parathyroid gland of less than 20mg will not be visualised by this technique. Earlier attempts to image parathyroid glands using thallium in a similar way has proved less successful than the use of MIBI.

⁷⁵SE SELENOCHOLESTEROL IMAGING IN CONN'S SYNDROME		
	UPTAKE BY ADRENALS	
condition	(involved gland)	(contralateral gland)
normal: after dexamethasone suppression:	normal none	normal none
adenoma: after dexamethasone suppression:	high high	none none
bilateral hyperplasia:		
micronodular: after dexamethasone suppression:	high none	high none
macronodular: after dexamethasone suppression:	high high	high high

Fig. 3.12 **⁷⁵Se selenocholesterol imaging in Conn's syndrome.** Adrenal gland uptake is shown with and without dexamethasone suppression of 2mg per day, starting early on the day of the scan and continuing for two weeks. High uptake is that greater than 0.3 per cent injected activity in an adrenal gland.

^{75}SE SELENOCHOLESTEROL IMAGING IN CUSHING'S SYNDROME		
UPTAKE BY ADRENALS		
condition	(involved gland)	(contralateral gland)
normal	normal	normal
adenoma	high	none
bilateral hyperplasia	high uptake by both glands or normal uptake by one and high uptake by the other gland	
carcinoma	no uptake or rarely normal uptake	normal or none
adrenogenital syndrome	high	high

Fig 3.13 ^{75}**Se selenocholesterol imaging in Cushing's syndrome.** High uptake is that greater than 0.3 per cent injected activity in an adrenal gland.

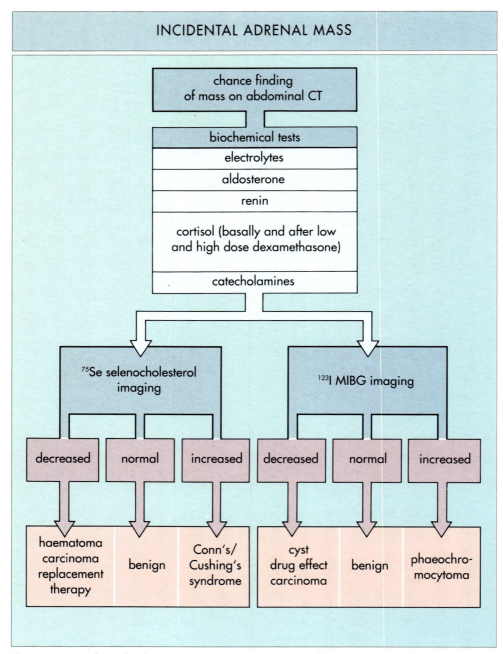

Fig. 3.14 **Incidental adrenal mass (an incidentaloma): a scheme for investigation and diagnosis.**

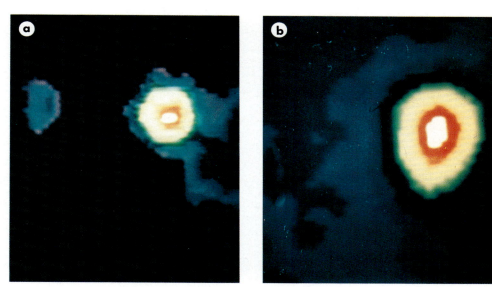

Fig. 3.15 **⁷⁵Se selenocholesterol adrenocortical imaging in Conn's syndrome and Cushing's syndrome.** Image (a) is a posterior view of the abdomen in a patient with Conn's syndrome (primary aldosteronism). It reveals high uptake of ⁷⁵Se selenocholesterol in the right adrenal cortex, shown in red and yellow, as compared to the normal uptake in the left adrenal cortex, shown in blue. Production of aldosterone by a Conn's adenoma does not suppress the uptake of ⁷⁵Se selenocholesterol by the normal adrenal. The purpose of adrenal cortical imaging is to localise an adenoma or demonstrate bilateral hyperplasia once a positive diagnosis has been made of Conn's or Cushing's syndrome, clinically and biochemically. A second use is to demonstrate whether an adrenal mass, seen incidentally during CT imaging of the abdomen, has a functionally significant abnormality. Image (b) is a posterior view of the abdomen in a patient with Cushing's syndrome due to a solitary cortisol secreting adenoma. A high uptake of ⁷⁵Se selenocholesterol is seen in the cortisol producing adenoma. In this case, the left adrenal is not visualised because of suppression of ACTH by the high cortisol level, thereby reducing the normal uptake of ⁷⁵Se selenocholesterol.

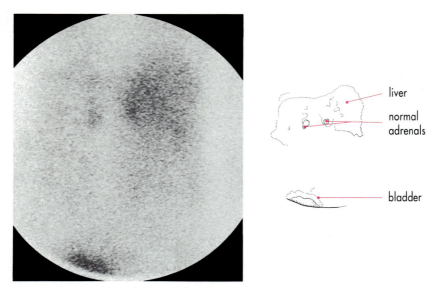

Fig. 3.16 Imaging of the adrenal medulla and neuroendocrine tumours with [123]**I**
(MIBG) meta-iodobenzylguanidine at 24 hours, posterior view. Normal appearance
of the liver and two adrenal medullae are seen. Radioiodinated MIBG has been used both for the
diagnosis and treatment of phaeochromocytomas, paragangliomas, neuroblastomas, carcinoid tumours
and medullary carcinomas of the thyroid. Due to its structural similarity to noradrenaline it is taken up by
the adrenal medulla and other tissues with rich sympathetic innervation, mostly via the neuronal uptake 1
system.

DRUGS INTERFERING WITH RADIOIODINATED MIBG UPTAKE AND THERAPY	
compound	withdrawal period (days)
inhalers, e.g. salbutamol and related compounds	1
isoprenaline derivatives	1
ephedrine and related compounds	2
noradrenaline and related compounds	2
fenfluramine	2
amitriptyline and related antidepressants	2
chlorpromazine, haloperidol and related compounds	2
guanethidine and related compounds	2
verapamil	2
nasal drops, e.g. containing phenylephedrine	2
reserpine	3
labetalol	3
phenoxybenzamine (high i.v. dose, not standard oral dose)	–

Fig. 3.17 A table of drugs that interfere with radioiodinated MIBG imaging and therapy. Recommended withdrawal periods prior to study or therapy are given.

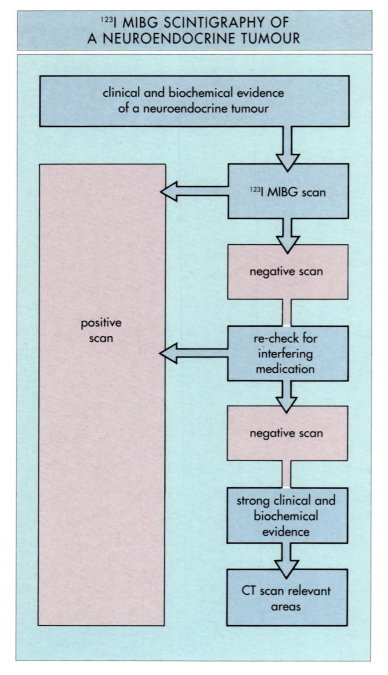

¹²³I MIBG SCINTIGRAPHY OF A NEUROENDOCRINE TUMOUR

clinical and biochemical evidence of a neuroendocrine tumour

¹²³I MIBG scan

negative scan

positive scan

re-check for interfering medication

negative scan

strong clinical and biochemical evidence

CT scan relevant areas

Fig. 3.18 Scheme for diagnosis of a suspected neuroendocrine tumour using ¹²³I MIBG scintigraphy.

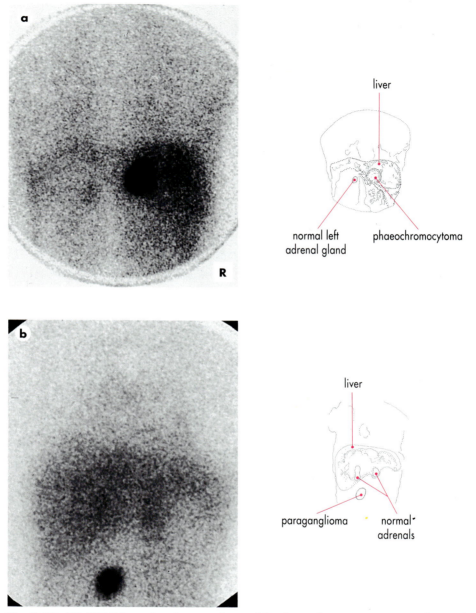

Fig. 3.19 ^{123}**I MIBG imaging in a patient with phaeochromocytoma and a patient with paraganglioma.** In (a) focally increased uptake is seen in the right adrenal region (phaeochromocytoma) and normal uptake is seen in the left adrenal gland. Note that the high levels of circulating adrenaline and noradrenaline have not suppressed the uptake and storage of MIBG by the normal adrenal medulla but cardiac uptake is reduced. In (b) high uptake is seen focally in an area in the upper abdomen, inferior to the liver. Uptake in the two normal adrenal medullae is also seen. This technique is 95 per cent accurate in the localisation of phaeochromocytoma and paraganglioma.

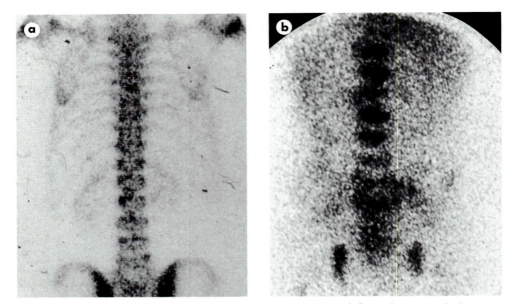

Fig. 3.20 Child with neuroblastoma; a posterior view of the spine. In (a) the bone scan is almost normal and the ^{123}I MIBG image (b) at 24 hours shows multiple sites of increased uptake in the marrow of almost all vertebrae and sacroiliac regions. [131]I MIBG therapy for childhood neuroblastoma is introduced after the initial chemotherapy and surgery for the tumour. Both complete and partial remissions have been obtained, but the therapy is palliative rather than curative.

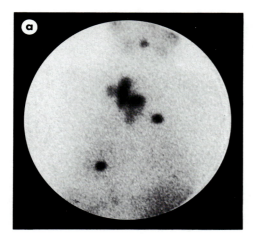

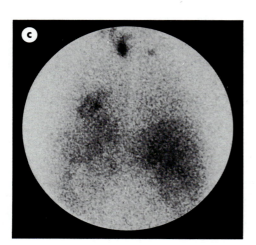

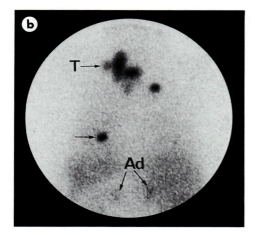

Fig. 3.21 Therapy of malignant paraganglioma with ^{131}I MIBG. The anterior view (a) of the thorax shows multiple sites of abnormal uptake in the upper mediastinum before therapy. During a course of therapy (b): after a total of two doses of 8.9GBq (240mCi) of ^{131}I MIBG, six months later (T; mediastinal tumour: arrow; lung metastasis: Ad; adrenal medulla). Image (c) taken after a total of approximately 37GBq (1Ci) of ^{131}I MIBG, five years later. The reduction in uptake is evident. Before therapy, this patient was incapacitated with symptoms and could not work. After therapy he resumed full-time work, was taken off of all drugs and has fathered three healthy children. In malignant phaeochromocytoma, paraganglioma and some metastatic carcinoids a good clinical and biochemical response is seen after ^{131}I MIBG therapy. There is usually reduction of active tumour mass observed on CT. There may be residual sites of uptake seen even though the patient is asymptomatic and catecholamine levels are normal. As the cell turnover in such tumours is slow, so is the interval to response. Thus, benefit may not be clearly established until more than nine months have passed and, therefore, a course of treatment must be planned.

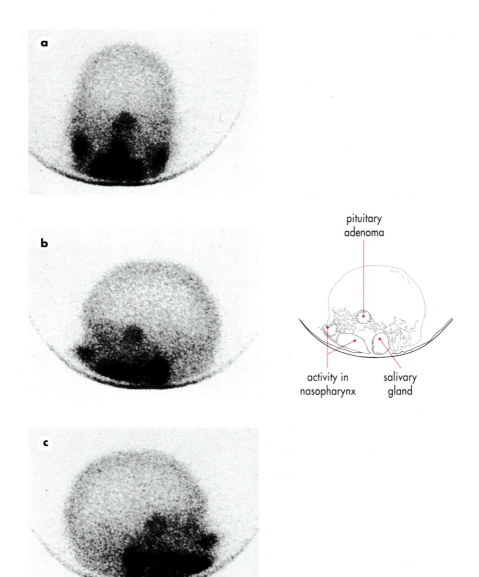

pituitary
adenoma

activity in
nasopharynx

salivary
gland

Fig. 3.22 Images in a patient with acromegaly using ¹²³I tyr-3-octreotide (somatostatin analogue). The planar images are taken at 10–20 minutes after injection: (a) anterior view; (b) left lateral view; (c) right lateral image of the head. There is intense focally increased uptake in the pituitary region due to the presence of somatostatin receptors on the cells of the tumour, which are labelled. Such patients respond to octreotide, therapeutically, with reduction in circulating growth hormone. Indium (¹¹¹In) labelled octreotide analogue may also be used for imaging.

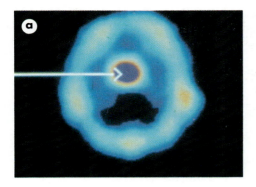

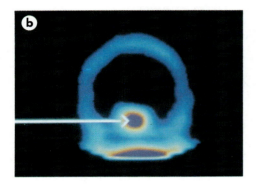

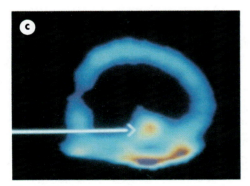

Fig. 3.23 Images of acromegaly taken with single photon emission tomography (SPECT) using ¹²³I octreotide. Image (a) shows a transaxial image through the pituitary adenoma, shown in red; (b) a coronal section; (c) a sagittal section also showing the pituitary adenoma (arrow).

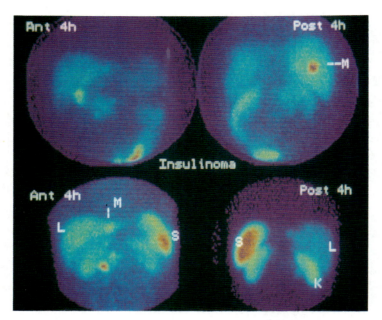

Fig. 3.24 Images of a patient with a metastatic insulinoma before and after chemotherapy. Images above are acquired with ^{123}I octreotide: the upper left image is an anterior view of the abdomen showing the liver outline with some activity in the gall bladder and gut; the upper right image is a posterior view showing the metastatic site (M indicates the tumour) in the posterior part of the liver. Below are images acquired with ^{111}In octreotide after chemotherapy. The lower left image is an anterior view of the abdomen showing the liver (L), spleen (S) and a metastatic site (M) in the left lobe of the liver. Some activity is noted in the kidneys since this is the normal route of excretion for this agent. The lower right image is a posterior view of the abdomen showing the liver (L), spleen (S) and kidney (K) Note that the lesion in the posterior part of the liver, detected with ^{123}I octreotide prior to chemotherapy (upper right), shows complete regression. A majority of gastroendocrine tumours have somatostatin receptors and can be imaged with radiolabelled octreotide. This technique can be used to image insulinomas, carcinoids, vipomas and gastrinomas in principle and to assess these tumours before and after therapy.

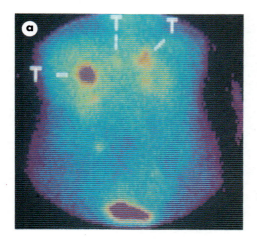

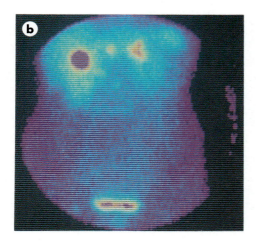

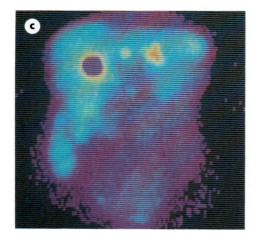

Fig. 3.25 Metastatic carcinoid tumour.
[111]In octreotide scans taken at (a) 10 minutes, (b) 4 hours and (c) 21 hours show uptake in the metastases (T). Excreted activity is seen in the urinary bladder in the lower part of images (a) and (b). Note that on the delayed images the target to background ratio improves.

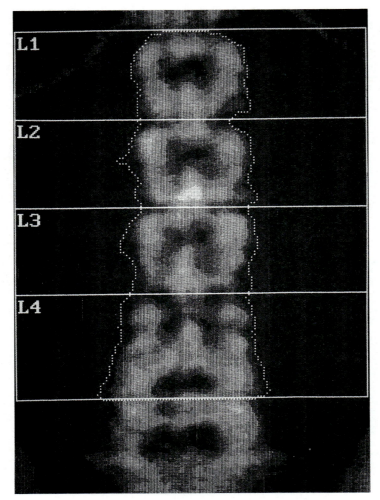

Fig. 3.26 Bone mineral densitometry measurement of the lumbar spine using Dual Energy X-ray Absorptiometry. The method is based on measurement of the radiation transmission of two seperate X-ray energies through a medium consisting primarily of two different materials, bone and soft tissue. The total bone mineral content of L2-L4 is measured in grams of hydroxyapatite equivalent (gHA) and expressed as gHA/cm^2. The normal range depends on age, sex, weight and ethnic origin. Bone mineral measurements from the lumbar spine, femoral neck and radius are used to assess the bone mass and predict the risk of fractures at these sites.

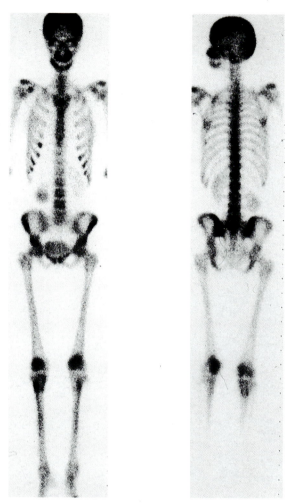

Fig. 3.27 Bone scan in hyperparathyroidism. Images were acquired three hours after injection of ^{99m}Tc MDP (methylene diphosphonate). The bone scan shows increased uptake in the skull, spine and long bones. There is also osteomalacia as shown by the symmetrically increased costochondral uptake. Bone scans with the use of ^{99m}Tc labelled diphosphonates provides a functional display of skeletal metabolic activity. It may be used in conditions such as osteomalacia, renal osteodystrophy, hyperparathyroidism and osteoporosis, to identify focal lesions, e.g. pseudofractures, vertebral collapse, avascular necrosis and generalised increase in bone activity.

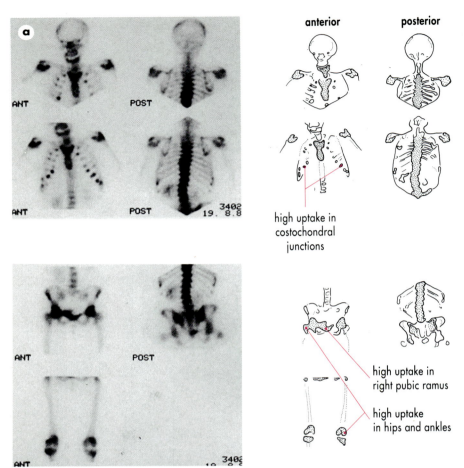

Fig. 3.28 Bone scan in osteomalacia. Bone scans before and after overtreatment with vitamin D derivatives. The set of images (a) show the following features of osteomalacia: the rickety rosary, symmetrically increased uptake in the costochondral junctions, increased periarticular uptake and increased uptake in the right superior pubic ramus (a pseudofracture). The set of images (b) show that overtreatment has returned all the above features to normal but there is hypercalcaemia, a feature of which is intense uptake of the bone imaging agent in the stomach. Renal uptake is also more intense.

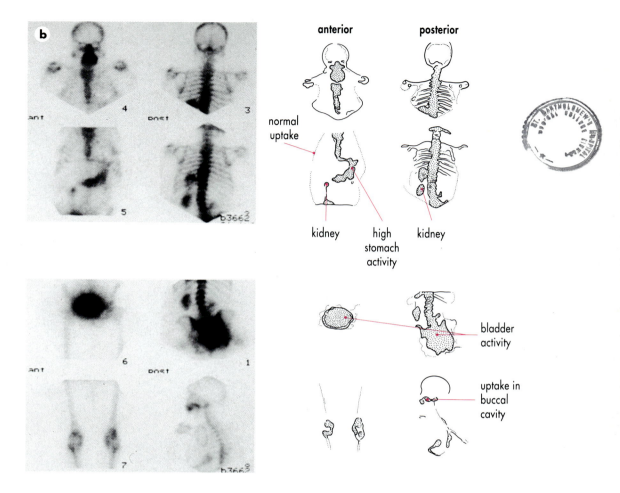

Fig. 3.28

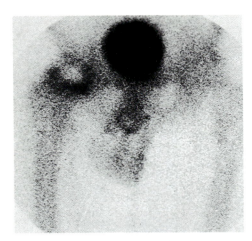

Fig. 3.29 Bone scan in avascular necrosis. There is high uptake around a central defect in the head of the right femur. Activity in the bladder and penis is seen centrally. The result is typical of an avascular necrosis of the head of the femur due to prolonged corticosteroid therapy.

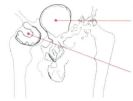

bladder and penile activity

increased uptake at focal defect in right femoral head

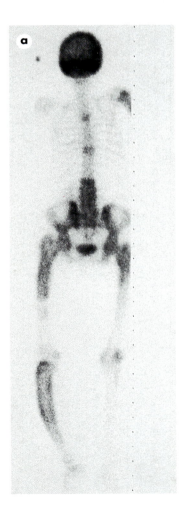

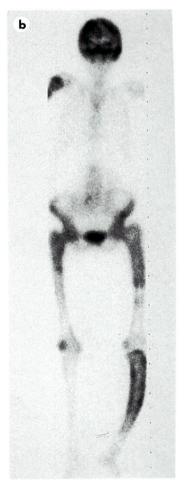

Fig. 3.30 Bone scan in Paget's disease. The ^{99m}Tc MDP bone scan shows high uptake in the skull, sites in the thoracic and lumbar spine, pelvis, proximal femur and left 'sabre' tibia: (a) posterior view; (b) anterior view.

RADIOLOGY OF ENDOCRINE DISEASE

1. Grainger RG, Allison DJ eds., *Diagnostic Radiology: an Anglo-American Texbook of Imaging. Volumes 1,2, and 3.* 2nd Edition. Churchill Livingstone, Edinburgh 1992: 2443pp.
2. Ross EJ, Prichard BNC, Kaufman L, Robertson AIG, Harries BJ, *Preoperative and operative management of patients with phaeochromocytoma.* British Medical Journal 1967; **1**: 191–198.
3. Siegelman SS, Gatewood OMB, Goldman SM, *Computed Tomography of the Kidneys and Adrenals.* Churchill Livingstone, New York 1984: 288pp.

IMAGING OF THE PITUITARY AND HYPOTHALAMUS

1. Ahmadi H, Larsson EM, Jinkins JR, *Normal pituitary gland: coronal MR imaging of infundibular tilt.* Radiology 1990; **177**: 389–392.
2. Chakeres VW, Curtin A, Ford G, *Magnetic resonance imaging of pituitary and parasellar abnormalities.* Radiologic Clinics of North America 1989; **27(2)**: 265–281.
3. Elster AB, Chen MYM, Williams DW, Key LL, *Pituitary gland: MR imaging of the physiologic hypertrophy in adolescents.* Radiology 1990; **174**: 681–685.
4. Goldsher D, Litt AW, Pinto RS, Bannon KR, Kricheff II, *Dural 'tail' associated with meningiomas on GD-DTPA-enhanced MR images: characteristics, differential diag nostic value, and possible implications for treatment.* Radiology 1990; **176**: 447–450.
5. Ostrov SG, Quencer RM, Hoffman JC, *et al,. Hemorrhage within pituitary adenomas: how often associated with pituitary apoplexy syndrome.* American Journal of Neuroradiology 1989; **10**: 503–510.
6. Pusey E, Kortman KE, Flannigan BB, Tsuruda J, Bradley WG, *MR of cranial pharyngiomas: tumor delineation and characterization.* American Journal of Neuroradiology 1987; **8**: 439–444.
7. Sherman JL, *Stern BJ, Sarcoidosis of the CNS: comparison of unenhanced and enhanced MR images.* American Journal of Neuroradiology 1990; **11**: 915–923.
8. Zimmerman RA, *Imaging of intrasellar, suprasellar, and parasellar tumors.* Seminars in Roentgenology 1990; **25(2)**: 174–197.

NUCLEAR MEDICINE IMAGING IN ENDOCRINOLOGY

1. Bomanji J, Levison DA, Flatman WD, Horne T, Bouloux P-MG, Ross G, Britton KE, Besser GM, *Uptake of ^{123}I MIBG by phaeochromocytomas, paragangliomas and neuroblastomas, a histopathological comparison.* Journal of Nuclear Medicine 1987; **28**: 973–978.
2. Chan TYK, Serpell JW, Chan O, Gaunt JI, Young AE, Nunan TO, *Misinterpretation of the upper parathyroid adenoma on Thallium 201/Technetium-99m subtraction scintigraphy.* British Journal of Radiology 1990; **64**; 1–4.

3. Fogelman I, *The bone scan in metabolic bone disease.* In: Fogelman I ed., *Bone scanning in clinical practice.* Springer Verlag, Berlin 1987: 73–88.

4. Fogelman I, Maisey MN, *The thyroid scan in the management of thyroid disease.* In: *Nuclear Medicine Annual 1989.* Raven Press, New York 1989: 1–48.

5. Goris ML, Basso LV, Keling G, *Parathyroid imaging.* Journal of Nuclear Medicine 1991; **32**: 887–889.

6. Hofnagel CA, *Radionuclide therapy revisited.* European Journal of Nuclear Medicine 1991; **18**: 408-431.

7. Khafagi FA, Shapiro B, Cross MD, *The Adrenal Gland.* In: Maisey MN, Britton KE, Gilday DL eds., *Clinical Nuclear Medicine.* 2nd edition. Chapman and Hall, London 1991: 271–291.

8. Lamberts SWJ, Bakkar WH, Reubi JC, Krenning EP, *Somatostatin receptor imaging in the localisation of endocrine tumours.* New England Journal of Medicine 1990; **323**: 1246–1249.

9. Ramtoola S, Maisey MN, Clarke SEM, Fogelman I, *The thyroid scan in Hashimoto's thyroiditis: the great mimic.* Nuclear Medicine Communications 1988; **9**: 639–645.

10. Reschini E, Catania A, *Clinical experience with the adrenal scanning agents Iodine 131-19-iodocholesterol and Selenium 75-selenomethycholesterol.* European Journal of Nuclear Medicine 1991; **18**: 817–23.

11. Shapiro B, Britton KE, Hawkins LA, Edwards CRW, *Clinical experience with ^{75}Se selenomethycholesterol adrenal imaging.* Clinical Endocrinology 1981; **15**: 19–27.